Northern Shaolin Style

Shaolin #8
Uprooting Step

Rick L. Wing

Jing Mo Athletic Association
San Francisco, California

First Printing

Published by

Jing Mo Association

San Francisco, California

www.jingmo.com

ISBN   0-9771648-8-8

Disclaimer

Please note that the author and publisher of this book are not responsible in any manner whatsoever for any injury that may result from practicing the techniques and/or following the instructions given in this book. Since the physical activities described may be too strenuous in nature to engage in safely, it is essential that a physician be consulted prior to training.

Dedicated to the memory of
Sifu Paul Eng
(January 8, 1941 - January 8, 2015)

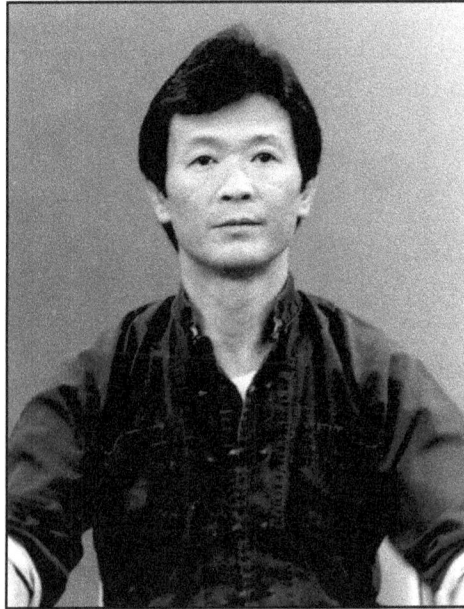

For his great help in translation and calligraphy in this martial series. He is a martial artist par excellence, a scholar, and a sincere, easygoing gentleman. He was a loving father, a devoted friend, and to his students, so much more than a teacher. He will be greatly missed by those whose lives he touched.

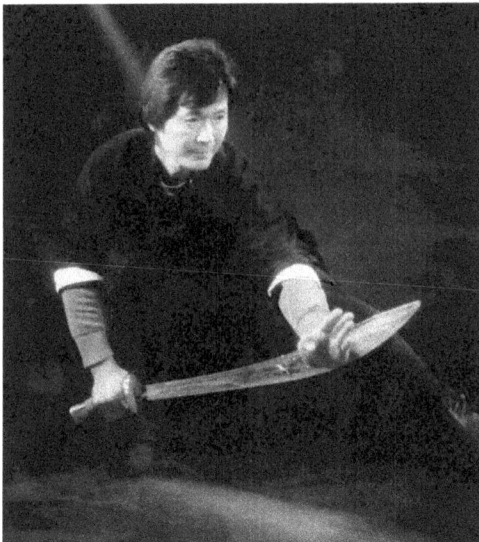

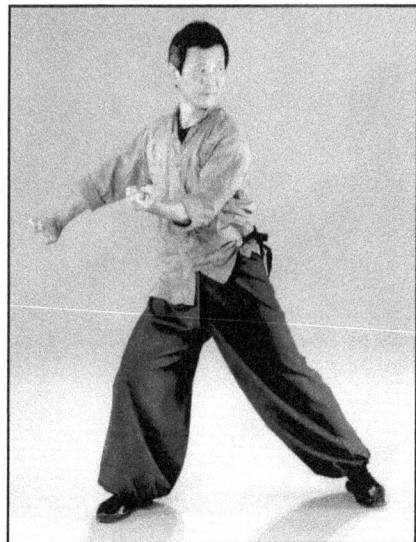

Preface

This book is about Shaolin #8, one of the five short sets of the Northern Shaolin Style. The set first taught in the system is almost always Shaolin #6, usually followed by Shaolin #7. After that, there is variation and many instructors will teach Shaolin #8, Shaolin #5, or Shaolin #4 next. This set teaches moves that are more difficult than the ones in the first two sets and extends the structure of the system.

I learned this set many years ago from Grandmaster Wong Jack Man, a top-level exponent of the Northern Shaolin Style. Many who have learned the style in the United States can trace their roots to this quiet yet profound man.

We hope that readers enjoy this book, and even if you have learned the Northern Shaolin Style from another instructor, hopefully, this book will still benefit you.

I have always wished to use the martial arts for promoting friendship between people.

To my fellow martial practitioners, with great respect.

Rick L. Wing
January 26, 2014
San Francisco, California

An Unofficial Biography of Sifu Paul Eng

This is not an all-encompassing biography of Sifu Paul Eng, but merely a sketch. I have known Sifu Eng for close to twenty years, and have known of him much longer. It has been an honor to know him, and I hope that what I write does him justice. Whenever I visit him at his studio, I always leave enriched by his extensive martial knowledge. His understanding of the art, any art, is deep and profound, with keen insight based on his knowledge of the Chinese classics on martial theory and, in addition, his rather amazing life experiences. His martial life has been an amazing journey; one that will continue for as long as he lives. His life is one completely devoted to the martial arts, and his skill and knowledge increase daily. Would that we could all do the same thing.

He has helped me greatly in my understanding of the style that I practice, Northern Shaolin, and he meticulously helped me translate all the names of the movements in the sets from Chinese to English. So, in essence, the "kuen po" (fist notes) I have created for the Northern Shaolin Style taught to me by Sifu Wong Jack Man is due to Sifu Eng. The task was a labor of love for both of us, and I believe all practitioners of the Northern Shaolin Style will benefit from our work. Our work was typically done on warm Sunday afternoons in his office, supplemented by perhaps six beers (Bud Light, to be exact) and maybe one orange juice or Coca-Cola. I won't tell you who drank what as anyone who knows us should be able to figure that out rather easily.

I spoke with Sifu Eng on Sunday, May 19, and Sunday, May 26, 2013, and gathered the following information. Of course, if there are any mistakes, unlike other authors, I deny all responsibility.

Paul Eng (Eng Ngok Ping) was born January 1941 in Hong Kong. Because of his poor health, his grandmother sent him, at the age of seven, to join a kung fu school in Hong Kong, thinking that exercise would be good for him. His grandmother was not knowledgeable in the different styles, and it was only important to her that young Paul go to a martial arts school, but not any one in particular. He ended up learning Choy Lee Fut and Fut Ga from Master Chin King Woon. Paul at this time was not yet aware of the concept of "style" in kung fu. Like most boys his age, it was enough that he was learning kung fu, and any kind of kung fu would do.

In 1949, he left Hong Kong and moved to New York, and for about two years continued his training under two instructors, Master Leung Hung (Yang Style Tai Chi), and Master Chan Kwong Ming (Choy Ga). Around this time Paul began learning of the differences between the various styles and methods of Chinese kung fu. He would often hear tales from the older students and even from Chan Kwong Ming himself, of another master, Wong Moon Toy (1907-1960) of the Fu Jow Pai (Tiger Claw System). Wong Moon Toy was a highly-respected master in New York Chinatown, and was also a member of On Leong Tong and Chee Kung Tong.

In 1953 Paul Eng and his close childhood friend Wai Hong (b. 1938) sought out the famous Wong Moon Toy. Although Wai Hong was about three years older, they were similar in stature and enjoyed many of the same things. Like two young detectives, they found an old ad in the Yellow Pages (Chinese), listing the address of Wong Moon Toy. They thought they would find a studio, and did not know that Wong Moon Toy no longer taught kung fu.

They narrowed down their search to one particular apartment building, and looking up from the street, they spied a tiger fork and Guan Dao on the second floor. They walked inside the building, found the apartment, and knocked on the door. They were no signs to indicate that this was a martial club, and they could see that it was simply a man's apartment -- not a kung fu studio. Luckily, Wong Moon Toy answered the door, but to the disappointment of the two boys, he said that he had given up the martial arts, was in semi-retirement, and did not want to teach anymore. Paul noticed that there was a large stack of Chinese martial art comic books on the floor of the apartment and since he realized that Wong was not going to teach them, he simply asked to borrow some comic books, saying he would return them next week. Tales of martial artists from long ago enthralled the young Paul.

Wong worked at a restaurant on Long Island about twenty-five miles from New York City, and as an employee of that restaurant was given room and board there. He usually stayed on Long Island six days out of the week, only returning to his own apartment in New York for a single day each week. Paul borrowed a small stack of comics each week, and dutifully returned them the next week. The young boys and Wong Moon Toy did not speak of the martial arts as that was assumed to be a dead topic. They had no expectation that Wong would ever teach again, much less teach them. For about ten weeks, Paul continued his routine of going back to Wong Moon Toy's apartment after school when he knew Wong was in the city, returning some comics, and then borrowing another small stack.

Then, one day, much to the surprise of Paul and Wai Hong, Wong, perhaps moved by the enthusiasm of the two boys, set up some tea cups and lit three incense sticks. In a short homemade ceremony, he had the boys bow three times before the incense sticks, once to honor their ancestors, the second to honor their parents, and the third (and last) time to pay respect to their new sifu, Wong Moon Toy. That being done, Wong then gave each boy a lay see (red envelope). The boys then began learning Wong's art in his apartment. The first set they learned was an advanced set, Fu Hok Seung Ying, followed by the northern twelve row exercise of Tam Tui. Both boys, now disciples of Wong, learned from him once a week and this pattern continued until he passed away in 1960. They had begun learning from him as young boys, and continued learning from his as young men. Since Wong Moon Toy was a member of On Leong Tong in New York, Paul Eng, like his teacher before him, also joined On Leong Tong. This was common among sifus and their close students.

Wong Moon Toy had been a member of the Jing Mo in Guangzhou, and learned from sifus Lau Jook Fung and Duen Yook Ching. Fu Jow Pai was a mixture of Hung Ga and northern style, and Wong Moon Toy was widely known to be a leading master of the style.

Perhaps Wong Moon Toy's affinity for the two young boys, Paul Eng and Wai Hong, may be explained by the following information about Wong's family situation. Wong Moon Toy's first son was killed in China during World War II during the Japanese bombings. His second son he entrusted to his good friend, Lum Jo (1910-2012), famed grandmaster of Hung Ga, in Hong Kong. Somehow, the second son died in a gang fight (the circumstances not clearly known), and upon hearing this, Wong Moon Toy ceased all communication with Lum Jo. Most likely, Wong Moon Toy held Lum Jo responsible, although Lum Jo himself may not have been involved with what actually happened. Most likely, Lum Jo did not even know what happened.

In 1957 Paul Eng and Wai Hong opened up their own studio in New York Chinatown where Wong would also come to teach. After Wong Moon Toy passed away, Paul Eng became Chief Instructor of the Fu Jow Pai Kung Fu Federation, and continued to teach in New York until 1965. His studio attracted many students and was very popular. His friend (and martial brother) Wai Hong was also an instructor at Paul Eng's Fu Jow Pai Federation. Cheng Man Ching, the famous Yang Style Tai Chi instructor, also taught close by.

Even as a young man in his early twenties, around 1962 or 1963, Paul earned the respect of the young men in his school. Because of internal strife stemming from kung fu rivalries within the school, there was much bad feeling among the members (not uncommon in many schools of kung fu), with the young men holding onto grudges and remembering all sorts of slights, whether real or imagined. Sifu Eng quelled their anger when he gathered all the students together, grabbed a knife with his right hand and stuck it into his left arm near the elbow. To this day, the scar still remains on his arm. When the blood began to drip out, he said, "I now take your pain. Does your pain hurt this much? It all stops today." With this act, the members ceased their quarrels and looked upon their sifu not only as a legitimate tough guy, but also as a fair and righteous man, and most importantly, someone to be respected. In their eyes, he was truly, "Sifu" Paul Eng.

One of Paul Eng's students also happened to be Kam Yuen. Although they were relatives, Kam did not even realize that Paul was a kung fu instructor and only happened upon Paul's studio by chance. Kam Yuen is now a well-known healer and was one of the teachers who popularized authentic Chinese martial arts in southern California in the early 1970s. Although Paul is only three months older than Kam Yuen, surprisingly enough, Kam Yuen happens to be Paul's uncle, since Kam Yuen is the youngest brother of Paul's mother, Kam coming from a family of eight siblings. Paul's mother is the second oldest of the eight siblings. Paul and Kam Yuen lived only three houses apart on Mulberry Street in New York Chinatown.

Kam Yuen learned from Paul Eng for about six months before he left for California to take a job at Lockheed Martin in Sunnyvale. Since Kam majored in Mechanical Engineering, it would be natural for him to begin his career by taking a job in the burgeoning aerospace industry in California. Kam's mother (Paul's grandmother) even bought him a 1965 Ford Mustang so that he could drive across the country to go to California. It was also known at the time that cars were slightly cheaper on the east coast, so it made financial sense to get the car before his trip, rather than having to buy one on the west coast (and pay more).

Although Kam Yuen was going to drive to California, it should be noted that in June of 1965, he only had a learner's permit(!), and so it was necessary for him to have a licensed driver in the car with him were he to make the long drive to California. Kam persuaded Paul to accompany him to California, and said that he would buy him a plane ticket back to New York if Paul would take it upon himself to make the long cross-country journey with him.

Upon arrival in California, Paul took note of the wide open space, the nice houses, the beautiful trees, and the mild and warm California weather. Paul did not need much encouragement to improve his English by taking classes at Foothill College, and, at the same time, extend his stay in the beautiful land of California. As things turned out, Paul ended up living in California… for much longer than he had planned. He never went back to New York, and Kam did not have to buy him that ticket for a return flight back to New York. Paul continued to teach Kam Yuen kung fu, and together they shared a two-bedroom apartment in Sunnyvale.

Paul and Kam frequently had dinner in San Francisco since it was not too far a drive from where they lived, Sunnyvale being only about forty miles from San Francisco. One day, while Paul and Kam were having dinner in San Francisco Chinatown in the latter part of 1965, they saw a Jing Mo Tai Yook Woey (Jing Mo Athletic Association) on the corner of Jackson Street near Kearny Street. Because of Paul's former connection with the Jing Mo Association through the heritage of his deceased instructor Wong Moon Toy, Paul became interested and went inside. It was there that he first met Sifu Wong Jack Man (b. 1941), a master of the Northern Shaolin Style. So, for $10 a month, Paul Eng became a student of Sifu Wong Jack Man. While there, he learned Shaolin #6, #7, #8, #5, #4, Law Hon #1, Hsing-I, and Wong Style Tai Chi (from the lineage of Wong Duk Hing). This rare form of Tai Chi Chuan was passed down from Ma Kin Fung through his student, Wong Jack Man. Although Paul had already learned the Tam Tui from Wong Moon Toy, he found Sifu Wong Jack Man's Twelve Row Tam Tui to have a better flow, and so, he willingly learned this set all over again. He came to appreciate the Northern Shaolin skills of the quiet Sifu Wong Jack Man.

Kam Yuen also learned from Wong Jack Man and, as a gift to his teacher, Kam gave the 1965 Ford Mustang to Sifu Wong, and then with his newfound earnings, bought himself a

Corvette Stingray. Kam Yuen learned Northern Shaolin and weapons from Wong Jack Man from 1967 to 1970. Kam also went back to Hong Kong in 1971 to learn Law Hon Kuen and more weapon sets from Wong Jack Man's teacher, Ma Kin Fung.

Sometime around 1966, Paul opened up his own school on 6th Street in Japantown in the city of San Jose. He had about eight or nine students, and among them were Ron Lew, Al Dacascos, and Malia Dacascos. Al and Malia learned from him for more than a year, with Ron Lew learning for a slightly longer period of time. Ron Lew, one of the very first to learn from Paul Eng in the Bay Area, learned the following forms from Paul: Tam Tui, Lien Bo, Siu Wan Kuen, Siu Lum #6, and Siu Lum #7, from the lineage of Wong Jack Man, and Gung Gee Fuk Fu, Fu Hok, and a staff set, passed down from Paul's southern master, Wong Moon Toy. Ron Lew, now a high ranking martial arts man and well-established in the arts of self-defense, Tibetan healing, and qigong, recalls, as a teenager, seeing Paul Eng working as a waiter in a restaurant, and because of the speed with which Paul set out the tea cups, Ron guessed that this waiter must know some kung fu. A short time later, he found his guess to be correct when he began learning authentic kung fu from Sifu Paul Eng in Japantown at the price of only $5.00 (a month!).

Paul Eng's kung fu training was soon interrupted when he was drafted in February of 1967 and had to enter the armed services. Paul, realizing that he would have to enter the army, recommended that Al and Malia Dacascos go to his own teacher in San Francisco, Sifu Wong Jack Man, if they wished to continue their study of northern kung fu.

Although Paul did not relish the thought of being drafted, he knew that his situation was not atypical of young men in the 1960's. After his initial consternation at being drafted, Paul accepted the situation and did what he had to do. This was the time of the Vietnam War. As a final favor for a personal friend before leaving San Francisco Chinatown for basic training, Paul was recruited by the relatives of said friend to give an "attitude adjustment" to a local bully who was also known to be a Wing Chun practitioner. Shortly thereafter, Paul left the city and entered the services of the United States Army.

Here is the long version of the story, a version which the reader will find far more interesting than the succinct version. Paul recalls that a certain family asked him to go to dinner in Chinatown. At the time, he did not know exactly why he was being invited. Near the end of the scrumptious banquet, one that impressed Paul mightily, the family told him that one of their members was being mercilessly harassed by a bully for quite some time. They then politely asked Paul if he would intervene, and perhaps give the bully a thrashing so that he would not bother their relative anymore. They then told him where "Mr. Chan" frequented. A few days later, the family gathered at one end of Waverly Place and pointed out the man to Paul. Knowing the man was a Wing Chun practitioner, Paul took no chances in the encounter. He would (literally) seize the initiative himself. He walked down the alley, up to the man and said, "Are you Mr. Chan?" Paul reached out his hand as if to shake it, and when the man offered his hand, Paul immediately grabbed it, yanked him off balance, tripped him, and pulled him down to the ground. He then mounted Mr. Chan's chest and began pummeling him in the face, perhaps fifty times (or more). Paul even began to tire from all the punching. Although Paul's hands were bloodied and bruised, he considered it a fair trade as Mr. Chan's face was now bloodied and bruised. He then left the scene, all the relatives walked away, and one Mr. Chan was left lying on the ground. The man's bullying had been stopped, the old-fashioned way. Paul then went to Wong Jack Man's studio on Pacific Street and told Wong what had happened. They both agreed that a good deed had been done and justice served. Wong then brought Paul some Teet Da Jow to rub on his bruised hands. Although the police looked for Paul, they could not locate him. He entered the military and went off to serve his country.

While in the army, Paul Eng became a Ranger and taught kung fu in the form of basic takedown techniques. He became a Chief Instructor of the Red Catcher Combat Ranger training camp at Long Binh in Vietnam. As Paul Eng explained, the techniques were quick and to the point. The timing was "one, two, take him down." Most of the methods consisted of arm-bars, sweeps, and takedowns. I inquired as to what the soldiers thought of the usefulness of hand-to-hand combat when they all had M-16s, and he explained to me the seriousness of practical combat and fighting in Vietnam. He actually bewildered me with his knowledge of military tactics -- the defensive perimeter, squad placement, claymore mine placement, machine gun placement, booby traps, night ambushes, jungle tactics, etc. etc. It was not easy for me to follow but I think I understood the general idea.

He explained that most combat actually took place at night, and during the day they would usually clean their guns, rest, or sleep. Depending on where they were in the field, he explained that nobody would sleep at night since that was the most dangerous time, the time they were most likely to be attacked or fired on. Sometimes, when on patrol during the daytime, the fog was sometimes so thick that one could not see one's own hand even if held directly in front of one's face. The probability of survival during certain firefights might sometimes be on the order of 50-50 (or even less). In one particular firefight, only twelve men out of forty (four squads) in his unit survived. Although his unit had set the ambush by laying out claymore mines, none of them detonated as the Viet Cong had cut all the wires as they crept forward. After the attack, Paul was one of the "lucky" ones and only survived by playing dead.

Paul was a member of "Charlie" Company, a group of around one hundred men, four platoons making up a company. The men of his company had heard that Bravo Company was caught in a night raid, their camp overrun, and the fighting came down to close-quarters hand-to-hand combat. Because of this, the men in his training unit knew that hand-to-hand combat training was invaluable, and their lives might literally depend on being able to apply the simple and basic methods they were taught.

Because a battalion had about 1,600 men, with only 400 doing the actual fighting (the rest in support), there was some downtime for Paul while in Vietnam. Although he was teaching fighting techniques to the Rangers, he also sought to improve his own martial skills while in Vietnam. For a few months (October 1967 to January 1968), Paul was able to travel off-base with the help of his South Vietnamese military friends and learn from the famous Chiu Chuk Kai, who taught Tai Chi Praying Mantis in Saigon. Although he only learned for a short period of time from Sifu Chiu Chuk Kai, Paul related that Sifu Chiu was kindness itself, always asking Paul if he wanted to learn more, and promptly teaching him more. Sifu Chiu understood that Paul's time was limited, given the circumstances of the war.

Then, in the latter part of January 1968, as Paul Eng so aptly put it, "The world turned upside down for a whole year." This period of the Vietnam War was known as the "Tet Offensive," and Paul Eng was, along with many others, forced to go into "military mode." He assumed his responsibilities as a combat Ranger, and referred to what he went through as "jungle combat duty." When I asked him what a "ranger" was, his short answer was, "Long-range recon. They drop off us off in a helicopter... they pick us back up." Paul had many tales of his rather harrowing experiences in the army, perhaps the most notable being when a large rocket projectile whooshed past him, missing his abdomen by about a foot. This rocket shell then slammed into a large concrete bunker behind him, completely obliterating the bunker.

He laughingly said that if the projectile came any closer, he wouldn't be around today, or there wouldn't be anything left of him --- he said one of the two things, but I can't exactly remember which. As for myself, I can only wonder... and imagine. He then related that the force of the projectile must have created something like a vortex, and he found himself about thirty feet in the air doing advanced gymnastics! Of course, at the same time that he was relating this story to me, I was thinking to myself, "Is this really possible?" and "I haven't had too many life experiences compared to Sifu Eng." Luckily, he landed in a rice paddy (if not for his "soft" landing, he may have been killed in the fall), found himself looking at the moon, and promptly fell unconscious. He later awoke in a military hospital. I hope that all of Sifu Paul Eng's students and grandstudents like the happy ending to this story.

In 1969 he was offered the position of Drill Instructor at Fort Ord in the United States but he refused. Instead, he went back to Saigon as a military policeman, and rose to the rank of sergeant, complete with his own army jeep! Ah, the beauty of belonging to the American military. He signed up for a second year as a military policeman, hoping to learn more from Chiu Chuk Kai, only to find that Chiu had moved with his second wife and son to Taiwan and was no longer in the country! If he knew that Chiu Chuk Kai had moved to Taiwan, he would not have signed up for a second tour of military police duty. Chiu Chuk Kai later moved again, and he stayed and taught in Hong Kong until his passing. Paul Eng later learned the majority of the Tai Chi Praying mantis system from the senior disciples of Chiu

Chuk Kai.

Upon being discharged from the army in 1969, a certain Sergeant Ngok P. Ng was awarded the "Army Commendation Medal" (September 19, 1968) for his outstanding service in the military. He also received a Purple Heart Medal, May 12, 1968. (And yes, that is the way his name is spelled on the official Army Commendation Medal certificate. I checked.)

He then returned to the Bay Area, with Sifu Wong Jack Man helping him to find a place to live on Jackson Street near Powell Street in San Francisco,. This apartment was very near where Sifu Wong lived. Many times he and Sifu Wong Jack Man would eat at Wong's studio on 880 Pacific Avenue, and they often shared meals together at the Ping Yuen Restaurant on Grant Avenue near Pacific Avenue. Of course, he also resumed his relationship as Sifu Wong Jack Man's student. So for a short period of time, Paul Eng lived in San Francisco, while Kam Yuen lived in Daly City.

From 1969 to 1971 Paul also learned Seven Star Praying Mantis from his uncle, Kam Yuen. Kam learned much of the curriculum of Seven Star Praying Mantis from Chun Jun Yee, a senior student of Lo Kwan Yuk and sihing to the famous writer and practitioner, Wong Hon Fun (Mantis King). Kam even had to pay as much as $700 to learn a form from Sifu Chun.

In 1972 both Paul Eng and Kam Yuen briefly became roommates again when they both moved back to Sunnyvale. Because many employees were laid off from Lockheed Martin in 1972, Kam being one of them, Kam decided to move to the Los Angeles area and teach kung fu. It was shortly thereafter that he began his association with the popular TV series, Kung Fu, starring David Carradine.

Also in 1972, Paul Eng, Kam Yuen, and Raymond Wong formed the Tai Mantis Kung Fu Association, "Tai Mantis" being short for "Tai Chi Praying Mantis." Earlier, Paul, Kam, and Raymond had all met at Wong Jack Man's kung fu school at 880 Pacific Avenue in 1969, and although they had offered the Chief Instructor position to Sifu Wong Jack Man, Wong demurred, and so, they formed their own association. All three founding members of the Tai Mantis Association had previously learned from Chiu Chuk Kai, with Raymond Wong learning from Sifu Chiu Chuk Kai in 1970. Sifu Raymond Wong first learned the My Jong Law Hon Style from the famous Yip Yee Ting in Hong Kong. Yip Yee Ting was known as one of the famed "Three Heroes of Hopei," the other two being Lau Fat Mang of the Eagle Claw Style, and Gan Dak Hoi, the "Monkey King." In China in the 1950's, the martial skill of these three men was so high that this was the sobriquet by which they were widely known. Sifu Raymond Wong, like Kam Yuen, also relocated to the Los Angeles area in 1973. Sifu Paul Eng remained in the Bay Area and currently teaches at his Tai Mantis Kung Fu Association in Campbell, California, next to the city of San Jose.

Sifu Paul Eng's knowledge is extensive as he has learned many styles from many different instructors. He has learned southern style as well as northern, striking arts as well as seizing arts, and arts which utilize strength as well as arts that utilize subtlety, and arts which emphasize hands as well as arts that emphasize the feet.

From Wong Moon Toy he learned Gung Ji Fook Fu, Fu Hok Seung Ying, Five Animals, Five Elements, the last two sets being the older predecessors of the more modern "Sup Ying," and the Iron Wire Set (Teet Sin Kuen). Paul learned all that Wong Moon Toy had to teach. Sifu Eng also knows about fifty hand sets of Seven Star Praying Mantis, thirty weapon sets from various styles, and twelve Two-Person Sparring sets. He also knows about ten sets of the Tai Chi Praying Mantis system, most of them acquired from the disciples of Chiu Chuk Kai as his own time with Sifu Chiu was rather short.

Although Sifu Eng has learned many styles over the years, his clear favorite is Seven Star Praying Mantis because he finds the movements to be flowing and the most natural for him. As he puts it, "It's almost like dancing." He can also intuitively sense the intent and purpose of the movements, useful for both health and self-defense.

Paul Eng has also taught Tai Chi Chuan at the Kaiser Hospital Physical Therapy Department in Santa Clara. I have always assumed that anyone who taught or practiced at a hospital must have some type of official certification, and as many of us in the kung fu world know, most of us do not have "official" certifications. Although we may study our art religiously for thirty or even forty years, many will not have any type of certification, at least not in the way one would expect in comparison to someone graduating from college with a BA or BS degree, or any type of degree for that matter. Let's say it this way, not too many of us graduated from kung fu university, although I do know that one can major in Tae Kwon Do in Korea. I would say that pieces of paper in Chinese martial art are more of a recent development.

So of course, the natural next question to Sifu Eng was, "How were you able to teach Tai Chi at Kaiser?" His deadpan answer was, "Oh, I got a recommendation letter from Bob Dylan." He said it rather nonchalantly, like Bob Dylan was just another guy off the street, so I assumed that this 'Bob Dylan' was someone who worked at the hospital or was some acquaintance in the medical field. I figured it couldn't be THE Bob Dylan. So I quickly said, "Bob Dylan? Which Bob Dylan?" He answered, "You know. Bob Dylan. The singer."

The singer? That's how he describes him? Maybe it's someone else then? I think to our generation, Bob Dylan was a little more than that, but maybe to someone who wasn't so interested in music the way we were, he was, perhaps, just a sound on the radio and just another singer. This is how he describes Bob Dylan? The singer? Folk-rock icon, superstar, master poet and musician, friend to the Beatles and Rolling Stones Bob Dylan. Voice of a generation Bob Dylan?

I was incredulous and dumbfounded, "Bob Dylan? You mean, 'Like a Rolling Stone' Bob Dylan?"

Sifu Eng replied, "Yeah, that Bob Dylan."

I couldn't believe it. "How did *you* get a recommendation letter from Bob Dylan? You *know* Bob Dylan? *You* know Bob Dylan?"

"No, I don't know him. Kam knows him.

"Kam Yuen knows Bob Dylan? How could *he* know Bob Dylan?"

"He taught a little bit to Bob Dylan and he asked him to write me a letter of recommendation."

"Really! Oh, really. Wow! Who would have thought that?"

So that was the end of that story, one of many from Sifu Eng. I can tell you this. I for one would have liked to have seen that letter!

One day, while browsing on the internet, I suddenly realized the connection when I went to the google search box and thought to type in "David Carradine Bob Dylan," since I knew that David Carradine of *Kung Fu* television fame was Kam Yuen's student. Perhaps that was the connection. In David Carradine's interview, he does mention learning kung fu, and introducing Bob Dylan to kung fu, via Kam Yuen. The full explanation now obtained and another mystery solved.

Somehow, I just couldn't imagine Bob Dylan as learning or even practicing any type of martial art, but I guess it shows that even superstars do things that regular people do. People like… us. As one can see by this brief interchange, talking with Sifu Paul Eng was always interesting, and always full of surprises. Of course, years later, when Sifu Eng recollected that event again, he told me it was David Carradine who wrote the letter of recommendation. So, it's one of the two, and I leave the rest to the reader's imagination. I won't fact check this one, and it's a neat story either way. This is the story as I heard it.

Looking back on his long martial career, Sifu Eng sees the most useful aspect of martial arts as being for health, and not for "kicking ass." This is something he has come to realize as he has gotten older, and something on which I must agree (as I have gotten older). When I asked him why he learned so many styles, he replied that, "All styles are good," and one need only find that particular aspect of each which can enhance one's own martial ability.

Truly, the art of kung fu lives in Sifu Paul Eng. He is traditional yet modern, practical and accepting of new ideas, and also a profound thinker in the ways of traditional Chinese martial arts. People like him do not come along often, and he is truly a martial treasure.

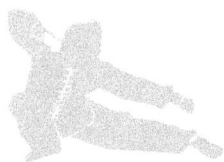

Table of Contents

Commentary on Shaolin #8

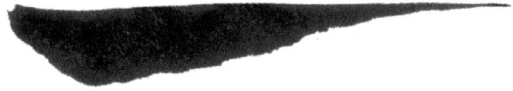

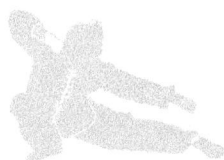

Commentary on Shaolin #8

Shaolin #6, "Close Strike," is the first set taught in the Northern Shaolin Style, typically followed by Shaolin #7, "Plum Blossom." Shaolin #8 was the third Shaolin set that I learned, but I have seen other schools teach either Shaolin #4, #5, or #8 as the third set after #'s 6 and 7. The order that the sets are taught is not carved in stone, and the order varies from instructor to instructor. All in all, it really is not a big issue, but there should be a progression from the simpler sets to the more complex sets. Sets #4, #5, and #8 are all above the level of difficulty of sets #6, and #7, but they are difficult in different ways. Some might say that #8 should be taught third because it introduces the leaping lotus kick, while others will say #5 should be taught third since it has the triple kick, a kick which links the double kick and the tornado kick by using a back hook kick in between the two kicks. Shaolin #4 is the first set of the five short forms that has a right front heel kick followed by a side kick with the same leg, and although this set does not introduce any new jumping kicks, it does have this kick which requires more balance since you are doing two kicks with the same leg without setting your foot down. Be that as it may, this book covers Shaolin #8.

Shaolin #8 is known as "Uprooting Step." The words, "bot bo," in Cantonese, or "ba bu," in Mandarin, signify the pulling of a plant out of the ground by its roots, hence the name, "Uprooting Step."

Here are different reasons why Shaolin #8 might be called "Uprooting Step." I can only conjecture why, as I have heard many different reasons from many different people, ranging from beginners, who know they are correct, and from instructors with decades of experience who have spent lifetimes in the martial arts, who aren't quite as sure. I suppose this is human nature and I shall let the reader dwell upon why this is.

One reason why this set might be called "Uprooting Step" is because the set has back sweeps, which "uproot" or unbalance the opponent, immediately followed by leaping double kicks. These movements would be #'s 7 and 8, and #'s 24 to 26. Another reason for this set being so named might be because a typical movement in this set is of an uplifting block followed by a hand strike. Moves that exemplify this would be, for instance, #8B, #10, or #27. In a more general sense, the set might be so named because there are many movements which the ancients thought useful in toppling an opponent by coming from below, such as #18B, which pushes the opponent from below by using a palm strike, or #32A which knocks the opponent off his center of balance by using a flying kick, or a technique such as #33 and #34, which have the practitioner throwing a thrusting punch while moving from a low cross-legged stance into an upright stance. Also, although the name "Uprooting Step" may not seem to be an aggressive or strong name, it actually implies that the techniques are very powerful, because to uproot a plant means that it will surely die as its roots will be exposed, and the plant will no longer have access to soil and water.

Another name for this set is "Three Palms, Eight Steps." This is not something I think that most practitioners would notice, even if they have been doing the set for years. This may be a figurative name; as it might prove difficult to see whether everyone's Shaolin #8 follows this concept of executing three palm strikes within eight steps.

Shaolin #8 takes a great deal of energy because there is a great deal of movement from low to high. Although the obvious example of this is the transitioning from low sweeps to high, leaping double kicks, there are also other movements which transition from low to high such as movement #19, which has the practitioner squat down and then raise up to a crane stance, or movements #22 to #23A, where the practitioner performs a side kick coming off a low twisted stance.

When I was young, I liked this set immensely because there seemed to be a strong "forward" energy. The practitioner should feel propelled forward by the various twists and turns and leaps and kicks. When I became older, I liked this set a little less because of all those… twists and turns and leaps and kicks. As I become older, I find that I tire more easily and that it is more difficult to exert myself to such an extent. Still, I must say that I know Shaolin #8 to be the favorite of the short forms of many practitioners in our illustrious art. On certain days, when I have the energy, Shaolin #8 is sometimes even my favorite set, although not as often as it used to be.

Another salient feature of Shaolin #8, assuming that the practitioner has only learned Shaolin #6 and Shaolin #7, or also the other short forms of Shaolin #5, and Shaolin #4, is the right leg back sweep, which is movement #7. This technique is rarely done and it takes time to get used to doing this particular movement. Another new technique is the leaping lotus kick, movement #20. Although this move is common in the longer forms, it only appears in the short forms in Shaolin #8, and this form allows the practitioner to develop yet another type of jumping kick. A technique of this type is supposed to develop the practitioner's leaping ability so that he can strike out with a lotus kick should the opponent be anywhere around him. Another new combination that Shaolin #8 introduces is the double kick preceded by a single kick, namely, the high front toe kick with the right leg. This is shown in movements #31 and #32A.

Another new transition seen in Shaolin #8 is that of the body spinning around to strike. As you are doing the set, note that these techniques are seen in movements #14 to #15A, and from #27 to #28 to #29. This is yet another way to strike the opponent, and it increases the maneuverability of the practitioner. This surprise technique, if used sparingly, may prove extremely unsettling to one's opponent. Spinning strikes, if properly timed and properly set up, are very useful.

Shaolin #8 also has, rather explicitly, an example of a seizing or control technique. In movement #18B, which is "Hawk grabs the shoulder," the practitioner learns to seize the opponent's hand and lock his elbow. Although the Northern Shaolin Style does have its share of seizing techniques, they are generally not emphasized in the forms. Oddly enough, the Northern Shaolin Two Person Sparring Set has a great deal of seizing and control techniques with wrist locks, arm locks, leg locks and the like.

Lastly, I might also mention that the particular way in which Shaolin #8 starts, with the left and right legs sweeping out and stepping forward, is also seen in Shaolin #'s 2, 4, 6, and 10. All the even-numbered sets begin this way, and whether this was by design or coincidence, I do not know. The way that Shaolin #8 ends, with its final movement of "Hero stands on one leg" and "Strike the tiger," is also seen in Shaolin #'s 1, 2, and 9.

Rules of Practice for the Northern Shaolin Style

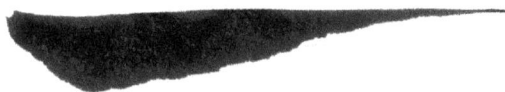

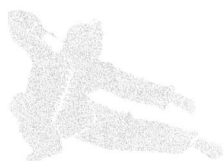

Rules of Practice for the Nothern Shaolin Style

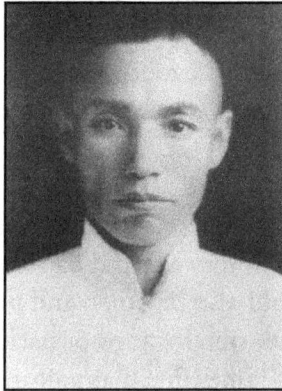

Gu Ruzhang

Editor's Note: This excerpt is translated from material originally written by Yu Pingzhang and Tan Fengya, former students of the renowned master Gu Ruzhang. The material was graciously provided by Sifu Paul Fung Ngar Tam, former Chairman of the Northern Shaolin Gu Ruzhang Memorial Association in the United States of America.

The Northern Shaolin Style is a very unique and special style. The moves are not flowery, rather they are simple and good for health. One will develop an agile body because the postures themselves require flexibility. If one looks closely at the style, one can see precise elements of attack and defense. This is one of the very best styles of Chinese martial arts. This style is an excellent vehicle with which to train the body and will. It should also teach one to cultivate good character. If this style is practiced, one can have the dual results of robust health and also an excellent knowledge of the important techniques and methods of self-defense.

As is important in any style, careful attention must be paid to the basics. Take heed of the placement of the hands and feet. One should know when to stand still and when to move through the various horse stances. Careful attention must be paid to footwork when advancing or retreating, or when jumping up or coming down. One must also know when to expand and when to contract the body. Be aware of how to use spiraling energy when one twists and turns while performing the sets.

It is important for the practitioner to realize that gains will come only if one practices daily without fail. A diligent practitioner knows this already. Only with daily practice will the skills become profound and the spirit strong.

The foundation of the body is the qi and the internal energy. Strong essence and energy will develop the spirit. According to an old saying from the Internal Canon of Medicine, "When the spirit is strong, the prognosis will be good, when the spirit is weak and dissipated, then the condition of one's health will be poor." Always keep this in mind.

The methods of the Northern Shaolin Style, like other Chinese martial arts, emphasize movements of the hands, the body, and the footwork. The eyes should be sharp and focused so that we may discern the opponent's intentions. The hands may be used to in various ways to defeat an opponent. The hands may be used to close him up, fend him off, hook him, or to cross the bridge and attack him. The body should be able to move in all directions with ease. This means the body should be able to rise and fall when necessary, quickly evade the opponent's attacks, and be able to lean forward and backward while still maintaining a strong sense of balance. The footwork should also be quick and precise so that when the opponent attacks one will be able to spin, bend, step forward or backward, jump high, or even flee at will. One must be agile while at the same time maintaining a strong sense of stability. One must also be able to discern the opponent's real intentions, and thus distinguish between his true and false moves. Do not be fooled by his false moves, and be quick to see his true intention and where the real strength lies in his attack. If you can do these things, know that you have achieved quickness of the eyes. This in itself takes hard work.

Be aware of whether the attack is directed to the lower body or upper body, and use the strength of the waist as a source of power. When fighting or practicing, also keep in mind the alignment of the fingertips, nose, and toes of the feet.

Keep in mind that the hands, legs and body together are capable of generating a great and powerful force which should be utilized in practice and in fighting.

When attacking or defending, always be aware that there will be a weak and empty side to the body. Just as when jumping up to double kick the opponent, realize that although your kick may be strong in offense, the other half of the body will be vulnerable. When one spins to attack the opponent, realize that although the spinning will generate strength and power in the attack, the other side of your body will be vulnerable and weak. When one attacks the opponent by leaping up and coming down on him; be aware that once the attack is completed, one may be vulnerable.

When one is fighting, the heart, being the source of emotional stability, should be calm like a mountain. The eyes should shine brightly like newly polished mirrors. The hands should reach out and retract as quickly as hands would spring back from an electric shock. The steps should be quick like a whirlwind and the feet should be light as a swallow skimming the surface of the water. The body should be as nimble as a phoenix flying and turning from side to side. One should be as stable as a mountain, but at the same time be able to move as fast as lightning.

Be aware of the six harmonies. They may be divided into the three externals, which are the hands, the eyes, and the body, and the three internals, which are the essence, energy, and the spirit. The six harmonies also refer to the unities of the eyes and heart, the heart and energy, the energy and body, the body and hands, the hands and feet, and the energy and spirit.

Lastly, be aware that the seven openings of the body, which are the two eyes, the two ears, the two nostrils, and the mouth, are very vulnerable to attack; therefore, careful attention must be paid to their protection. If the eyes are hurt, this will harm the Qingming point, which is related to the liver. If the ears are hurt, this will harm the Hui and the Tinghui points, which are related to the kidney and lung meridians. If the nostrils (or the nose) are hurt, this will cause injury to the Sujiao and Yingxiang points, which are related to the lung meridians. If the mouth is hurt, this will cause injury to the spleen and heart meridians. It is vital that these openings be well protected at all times.

Editor's Note: The above words are clearly very detailed and give excellent advice regarding the practice of Northern Shaolin. I myself am not able to keep all these things in mind while practicing, and I find that I can keep only a few things in mind. I try to keep my upper body relaxed and utilize strength only when absolutely necessary, preferring to concentrate the power at the last possible moment. I use a low horse for exercise and health purposes, and a high horse for speed and rapidity of movement. I do not like to stop and hold positions for very long because I do not like to pose and find this is not very useful if I will be forced to use the martial arts for self-defense. I prefer to look only in a general direction but try not to focus on anything in particular. In general, it is good to push one's body to its higher limits so as to achieve maximum potential. Also, extend the limbs so that the muscles will become loose yet strong. In physical confrontation, keep a calm heart and try not to be afraid, but at the same time, do not underestimate your adversary. This is advice that my teacher gave to me. Everything should fall into place if one does these things. I write these things down so that I will not have to overly repeat them to my students, and also so that I myself can keep them in mind.

Shaolin #8: Uprooting Step - The Form

拔步

北派少林拳

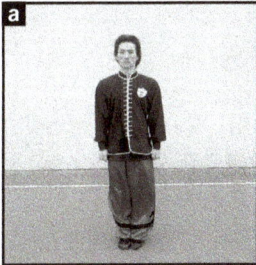

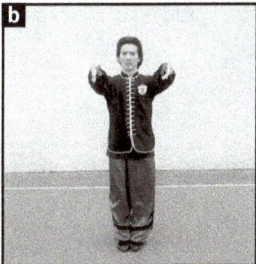

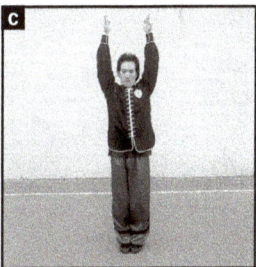

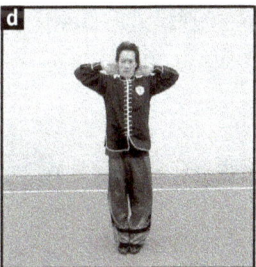

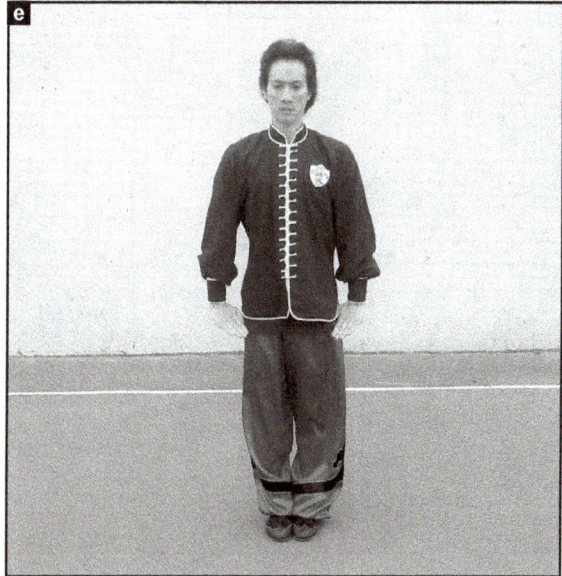

Opening position

The Salute: Stand at attention with fists at your sides. In one continuous motion, raise your hands up, and then push down with both palms. This is the Northern Shaolin salute.

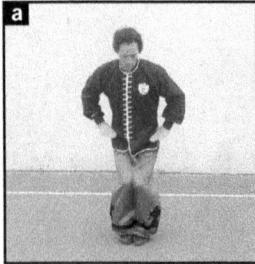

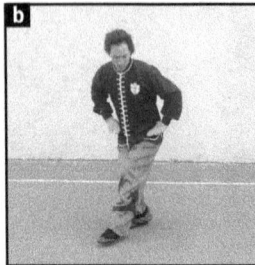

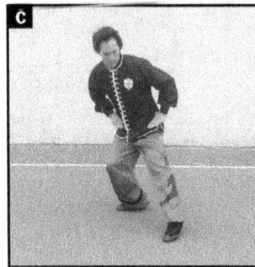

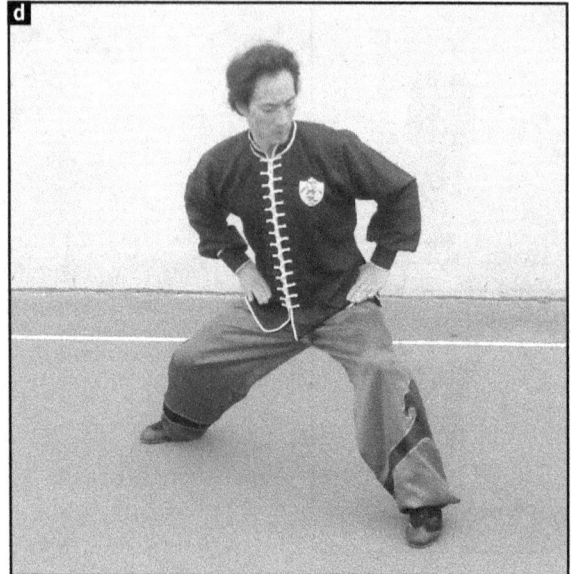

一、仙人彈衣上

1A - Immortal shakes his clothes. Step forward.

Step out and to your left with the left leg and trace a counter-clockwise circular shape on the floor. Put the weight on the left leg.

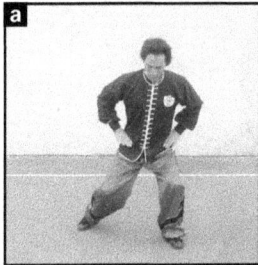

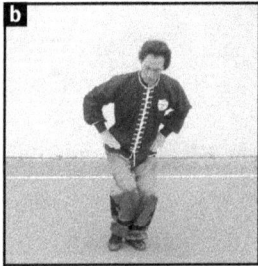

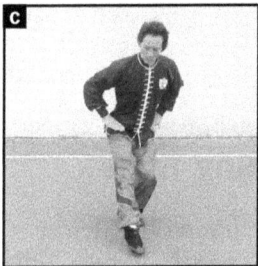

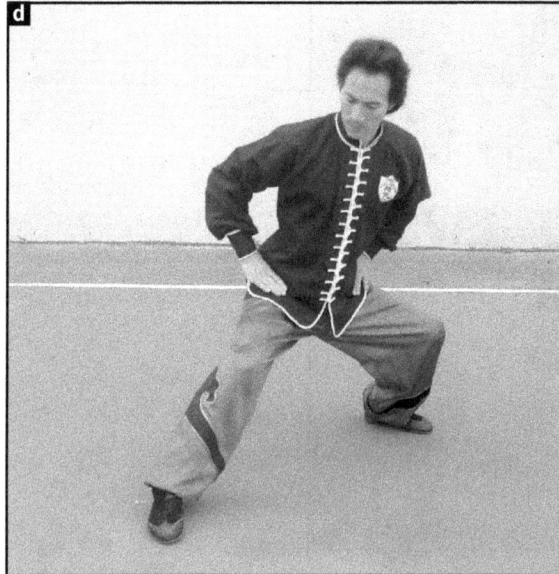

一、上步

1B - Step forward.

Now, with the right foot, trace a clockwise circular shape on the floor by first bringing the right foot alongside the left foot, and then forward and to the right in one continuous motion.

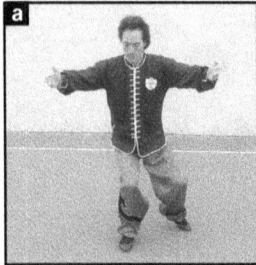

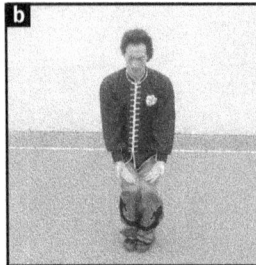

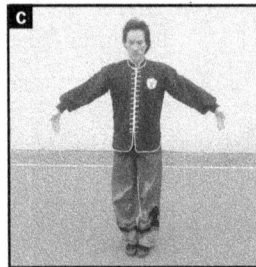

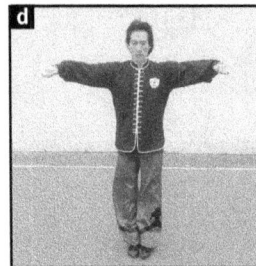

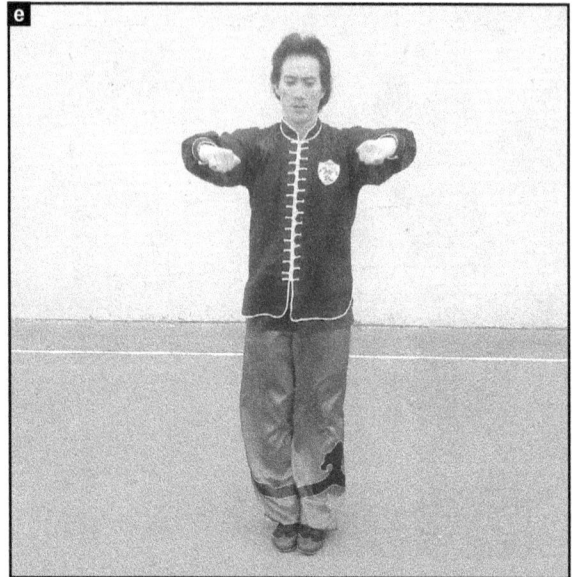

一、對拳

1C - Double matching fists.

As you bring the left foot alongside the right foot, bring the hands forward, palms up, and bend your knees slightly.

As you dip down and bend your knees slightly, brush the backs of both hands against the top of your thighs.

Then bring both hands forward in a circular motion forming fists with both hands. Your hands should be held at approximately chest level.

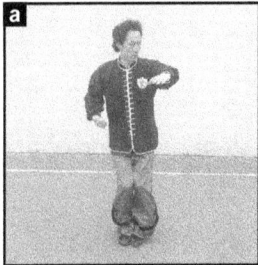

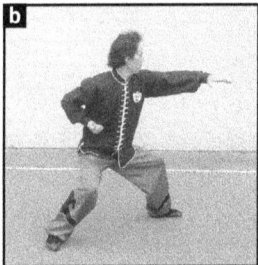

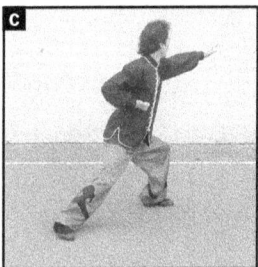

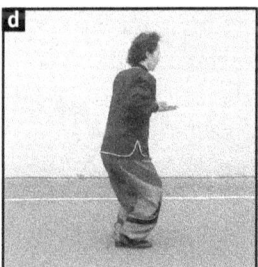

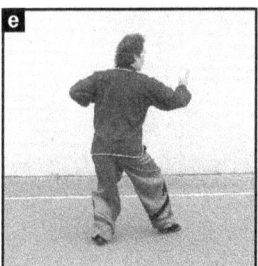

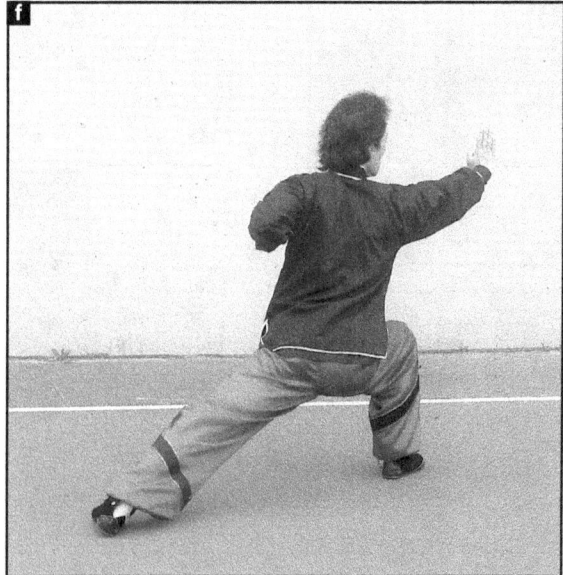

二、摟 手 斜 步 右 切 掌

2 - (Left) Pulling Hand. Angled side) step. Advance with a (right) cutting palm in a right bow stance.

Step back and to your left at a 45 degree angle with the left foot, and at the same time make a counterclockwise clearing motion from right to left with your left hand.

As you close your left hand into a fist, step up with the right leg into a right bow stance and strike with the blade edge of your palm.

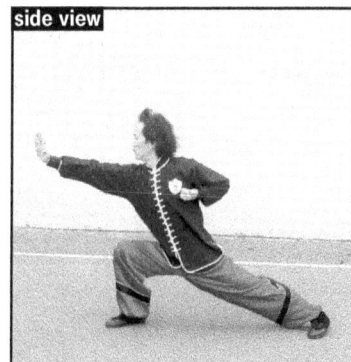

side view

19

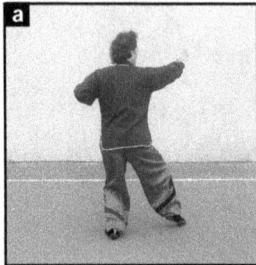

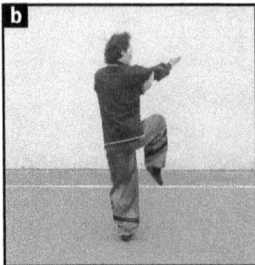

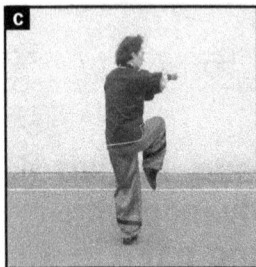

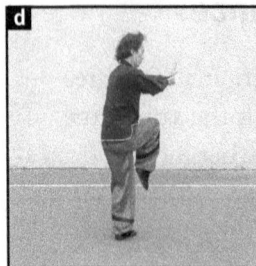

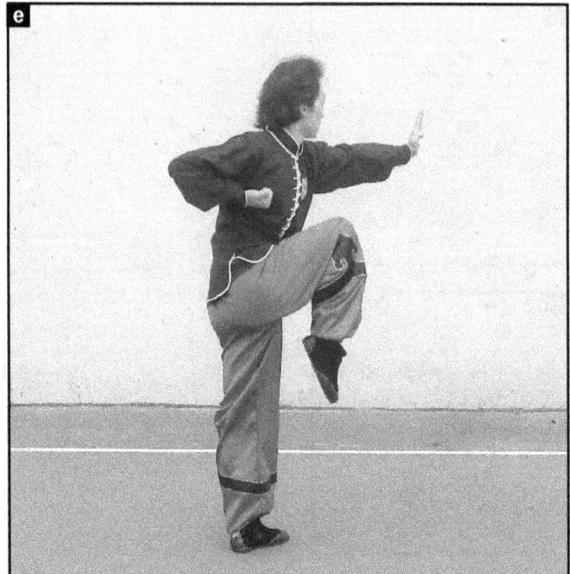

三、撤 步

3A - Step back. (Right leg up, left palm).

Withdraw your right leg and raise your right leg to a crane stance while wiping the back of the left hand along the outside of the right arm. Withdraw the right fist and push out with the edge of the left palm. (Alternatively, some may wish to wipe the inside of the left palm along the inside of the right arm. Either is acceptable.)

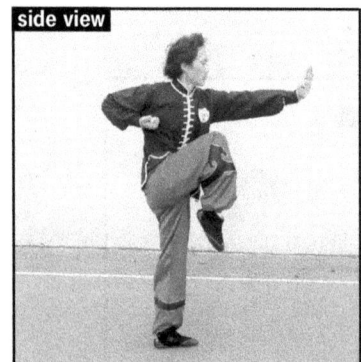

side view

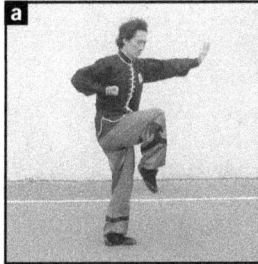

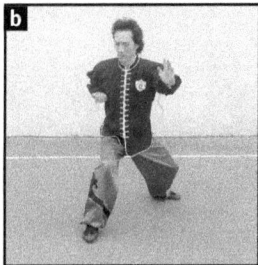

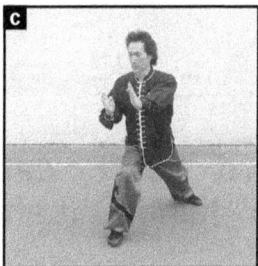

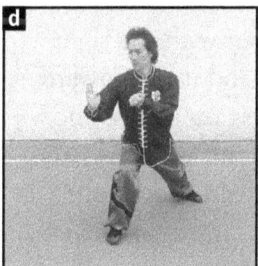

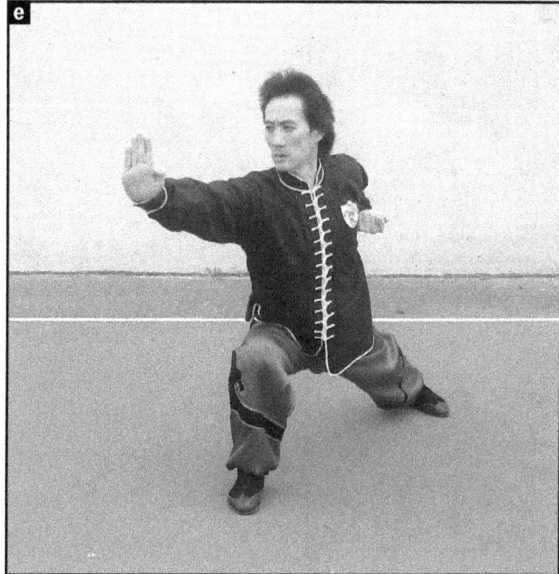

三、 撩陰掌

3B - "Uppercut to the groin" (right) palm strike.

Pivot on the left foot and turning towards your right, face the opposite direction. Step down with the right leg into a right bow stance and strike with the blade edge of the right palm. Your right foot is at a 45-degree angle from the left foot.

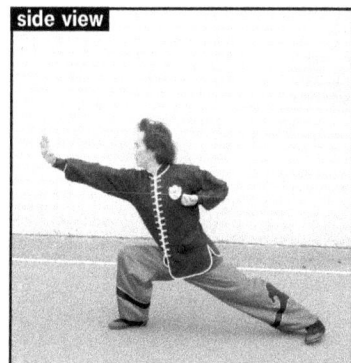

side view

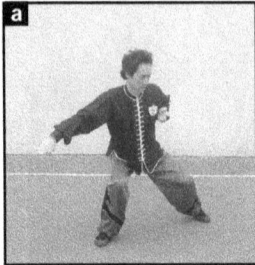

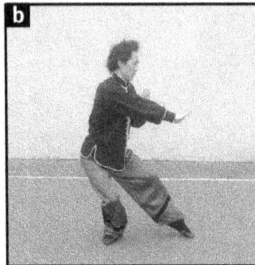

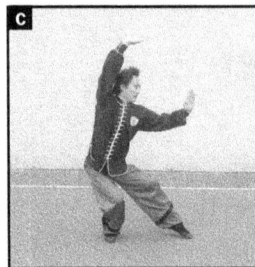

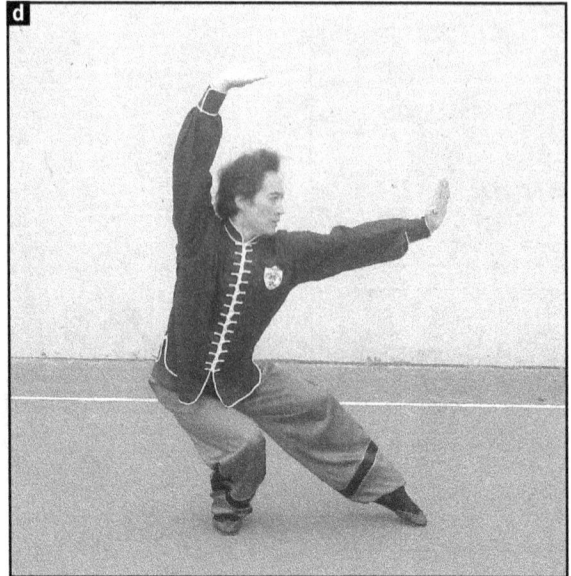

四、 撩 手 上 步

4A - Step forward (Left cat stance). Lift hands. (Left palm strike).

Lightly stamp the floor with the right foot and move the right hand in an upward clockwise circle. Sit in a left cat stance and push out with the edge of the left palm. Your right hand is open and is held above your head.

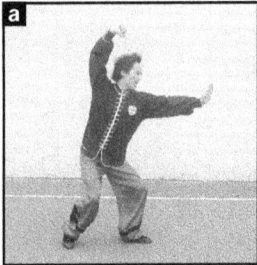

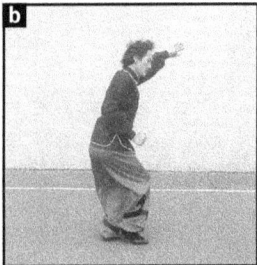

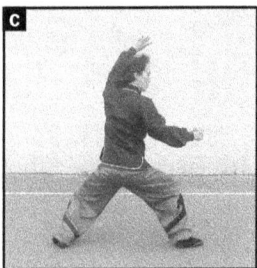

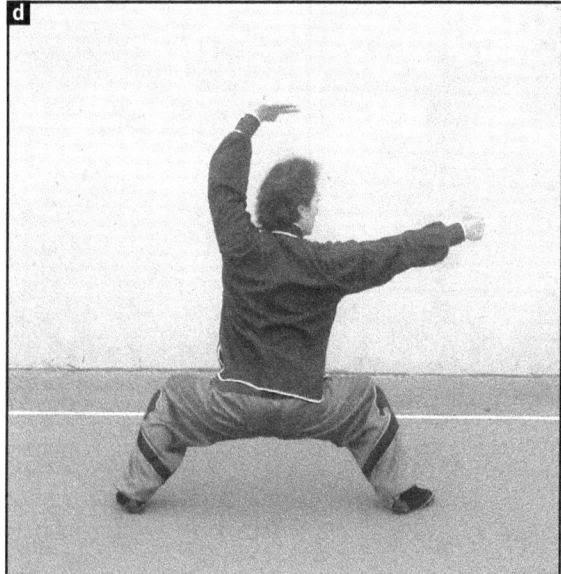

四、坐馬架打式

4B - Sit in horse stance. Block and strike. (Right fist strike).

Step down with your left foot and bring the right foot forward past your left foot into a horse stance with the right foot now forward. As you bring the right foot forward, block down with an open left hand and strike directly forward with a right vertical fist.

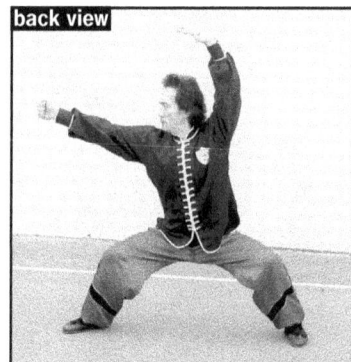

back view

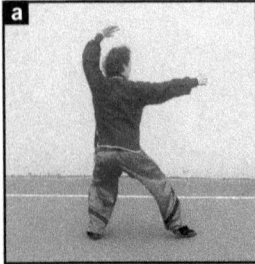

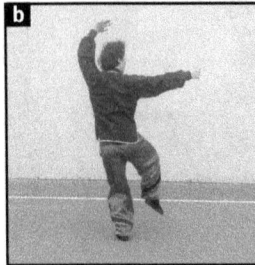

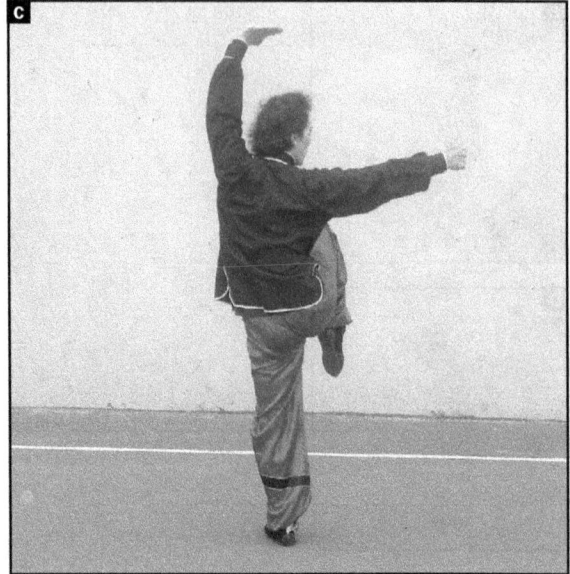

五、震足纏手上步壓打

5A - Raise the right leg.

Withdraw and lift the right leg into a crane stance. You can either point the toe of the right foot downward, or you can leave the foot level and flex it slightly upward. Either way is acceptable.

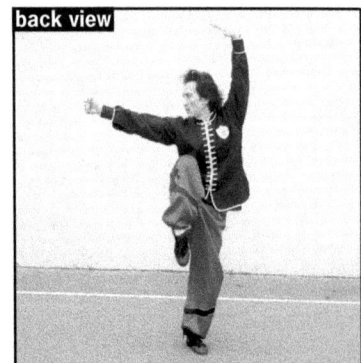

back view

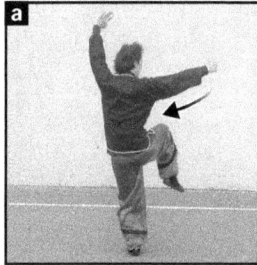

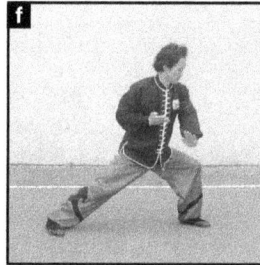

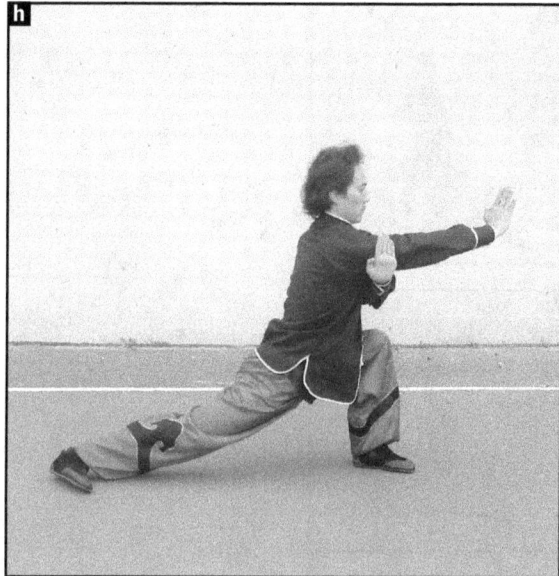

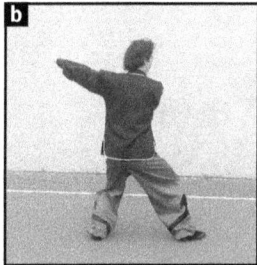

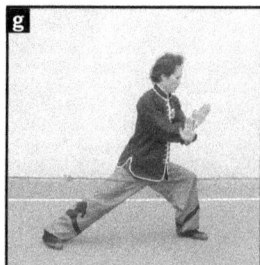

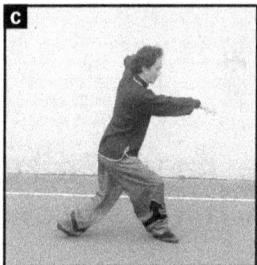

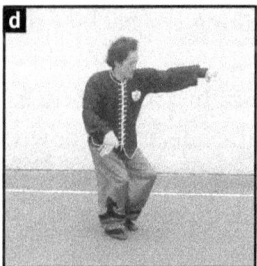

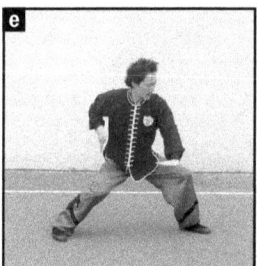

五、 震 足 纏 手 上 步 壓 打

5B - Stamp the foot. Tangling hand. Step forward. Press and strike.

Then, step down with the right leg and withdraw the right hand. The right hand will make a clockwise circular motion followed by the left hand.

As you step forward into a left bow stance, strike directly forward with the blade edge of the right palm. The back of the left hand will be placed alongside the right tricep.

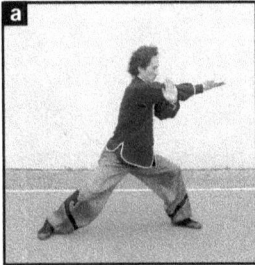

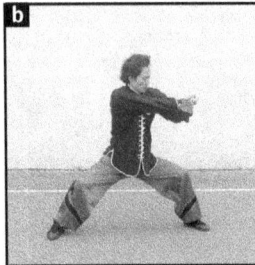

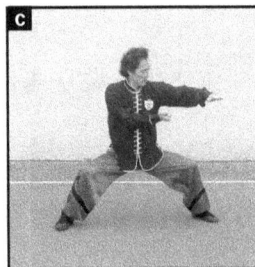

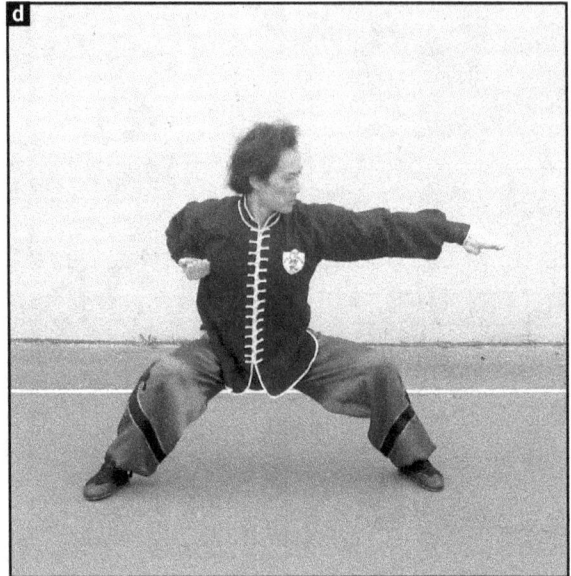

六、 脱手撑掌坐馬式

6 - Wipe off the hand. Strike with the palm. Horse stance.

As you withdraw into a horse stance, slide the back of the left hand along the back of the right arm.

As you withdraw the right arm and tuck the right fist in at your right side, strike down and directly in front of you with the blade edge of the left palm. The left palm is now facing downward.

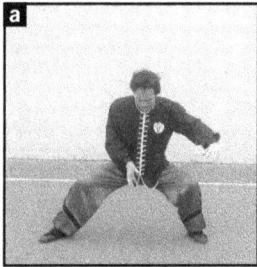

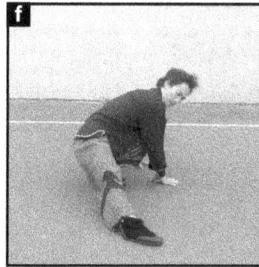

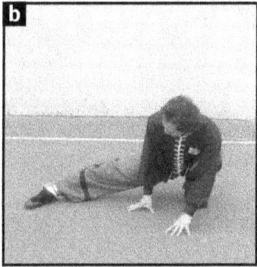

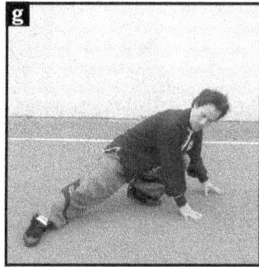

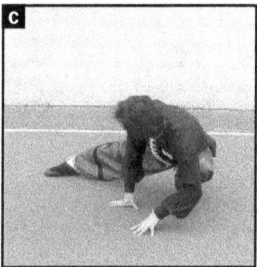

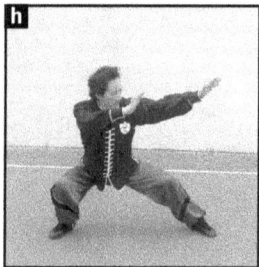

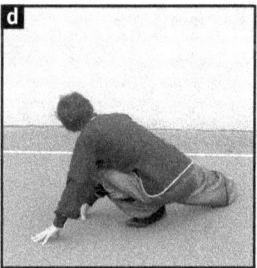

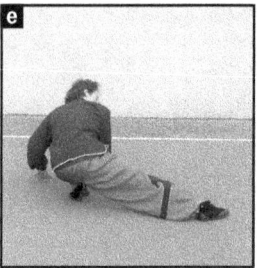

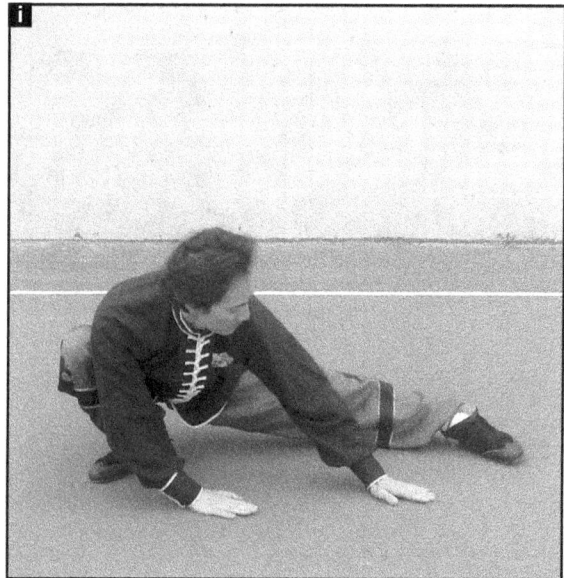

七、 後 掃 堂 拍 地 飛 沙

7 - Back sweep. Slap the ground. Flying sand.

Put the weight on your left leg and turn towards your right. Place your hands on the floor and perform a back sweep with the right leg.

Slap the ground with both hands as you sit down in a left scattered stance. You may slap the ground with force if so desired.

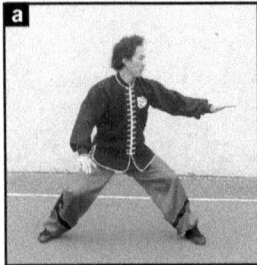

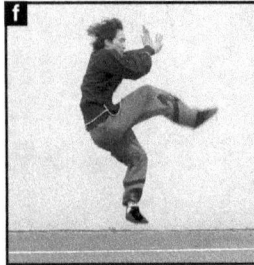

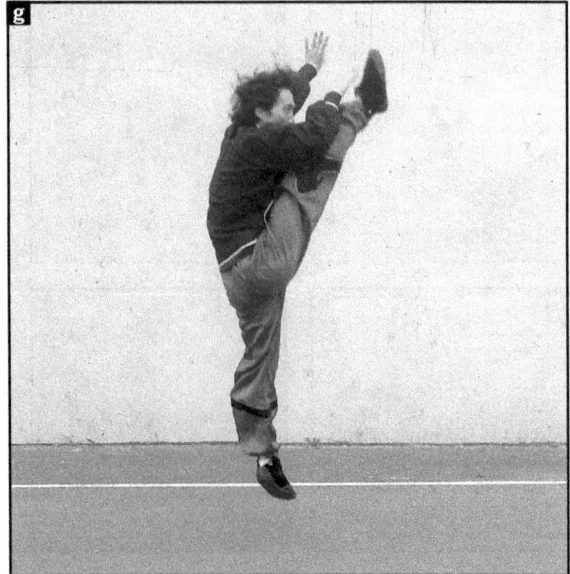

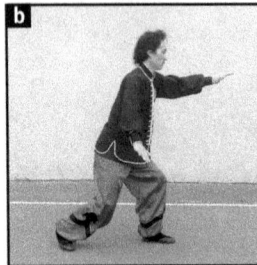

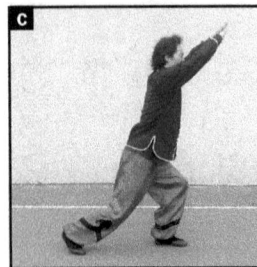

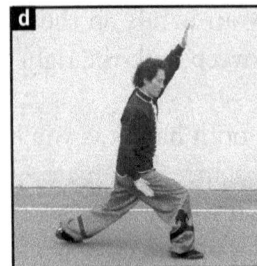

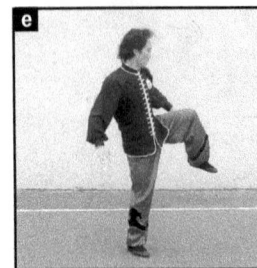

八、 二 起 腿

8A - Double kick.

Rise up, and run directly forward and do a right leg double kick, slapping the instep of the right foot with the right hand.

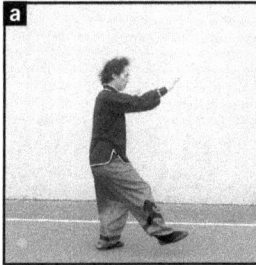

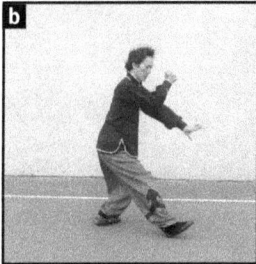

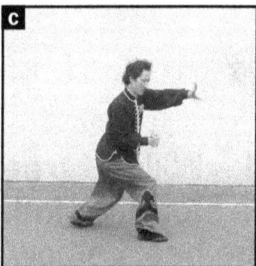

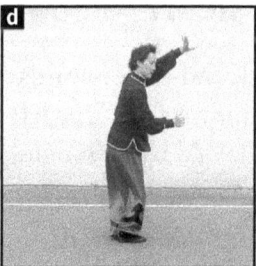

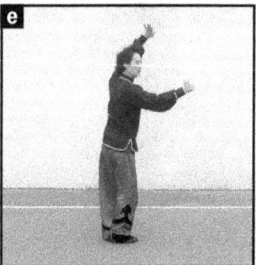

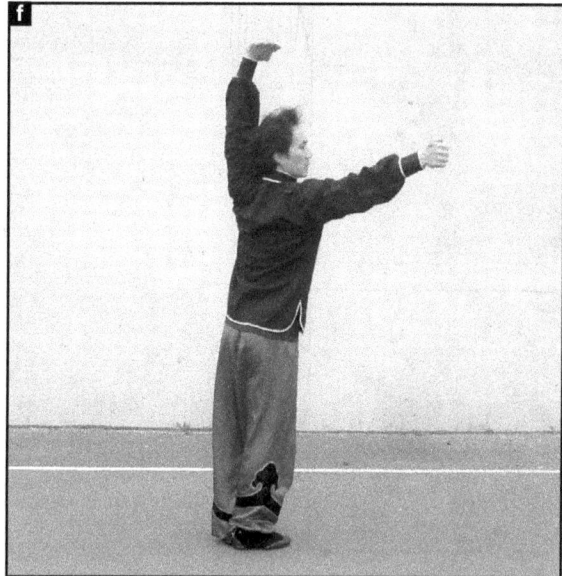

八、 直立架打式

8B - Stand up. Block and strike.

Step down with the right foot at a 45-degree angle to your left foot and, as you bring your left foot alongside your right foot, block upward in a counter-clockwise clearing motion with the open left hand, and then strike with a right vertical fist. Both feet are now together.

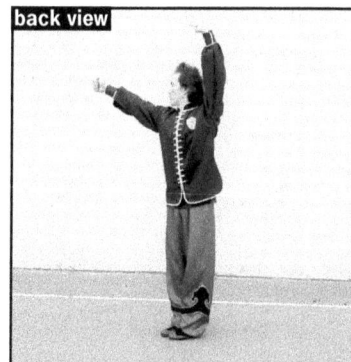

back view

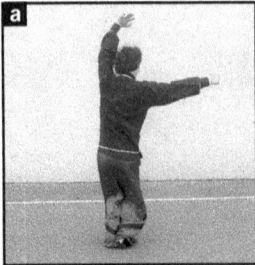

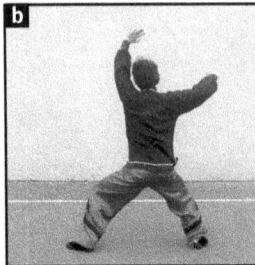

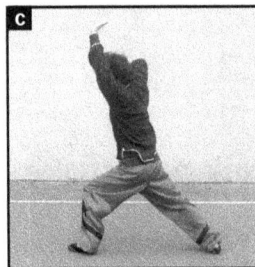

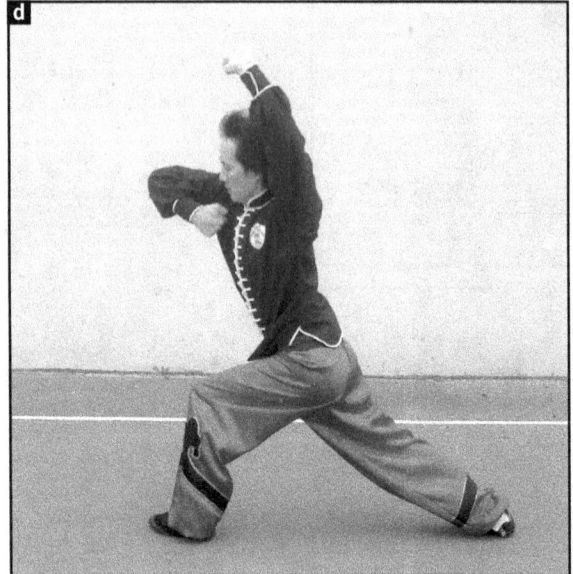

九、 回身迎風擺柳窩心肘

9 - Turn around. Willow tree swaying in the blowing wind. Go through the heart elbow. ("Protect the heart" elbow).

Step the left foot back and turn towards your left. Shift into a left bow stance. The left hand will block down, followed by a swinging downward right elbow strike.

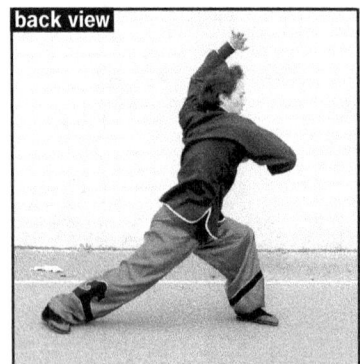

back view

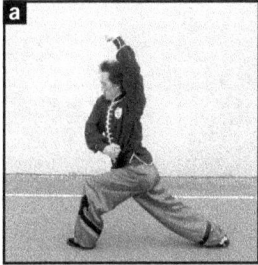

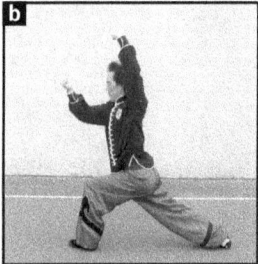

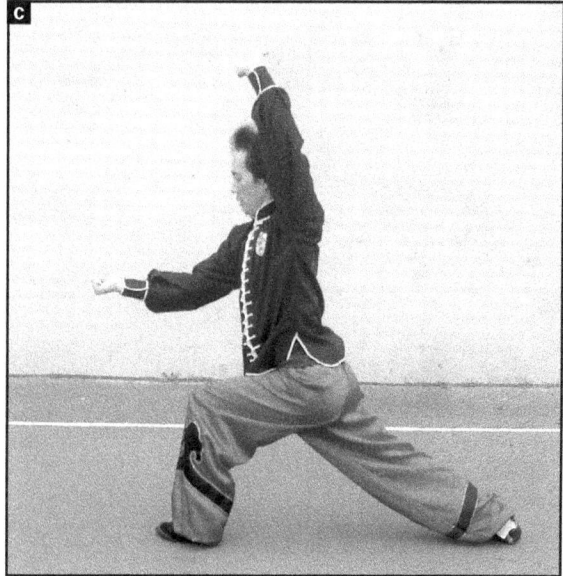

十、扎拳

10A - Strike with the fist.
(Backfist strike).

Then unwind the right fist using an upward clockwise motion so as to strike with the right backfist.

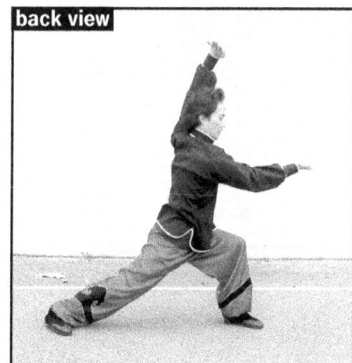

back view

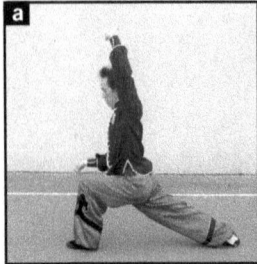

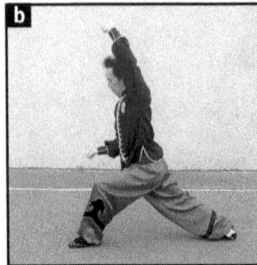

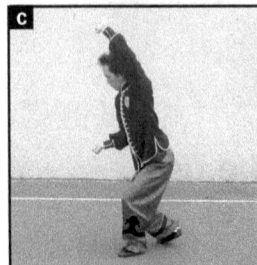

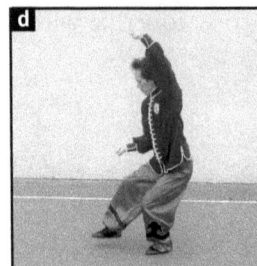

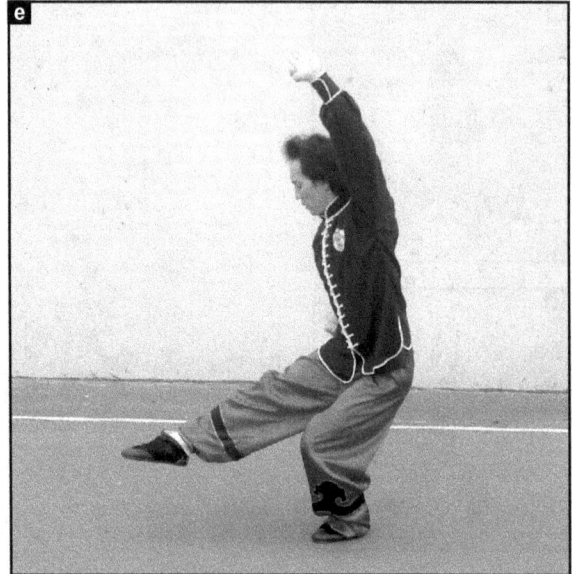

十、踢脚

10B - Kick with the (right) leg.

Turn the left foot slightly to the left and then kick forward at a low level with the right leg using the toe. As you kick out with the right leg, pull the right arm back and withdraw the right fist to the side of the waist.

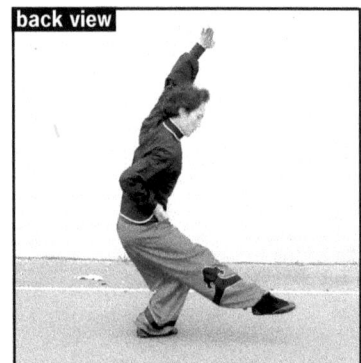
back view

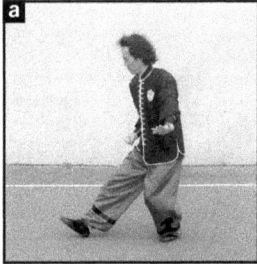

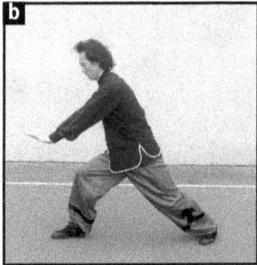

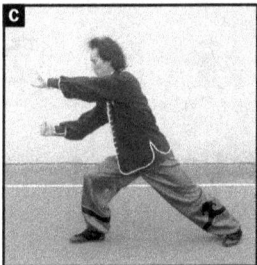

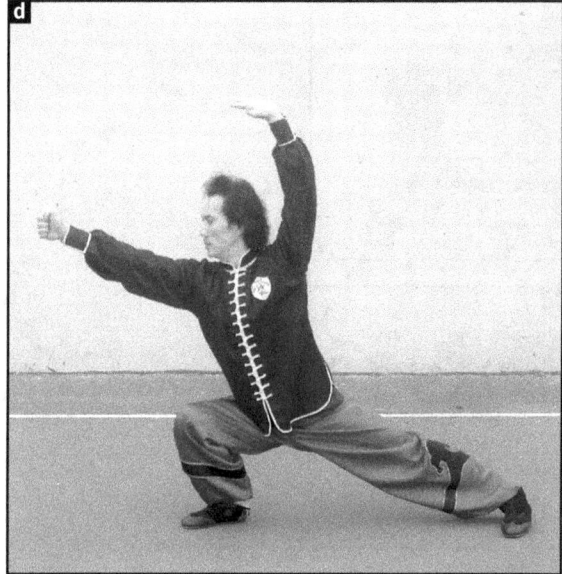

十、弓步架打式

10C - Forward stance. Block and strike. (Right fist).

Step forward into a right bow stance and strike directly forward with a right vertical fist.

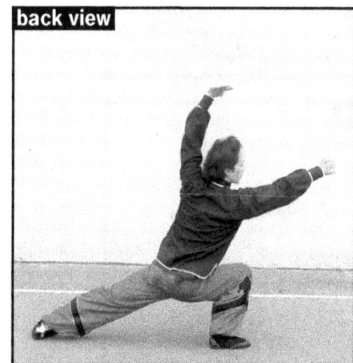

back view

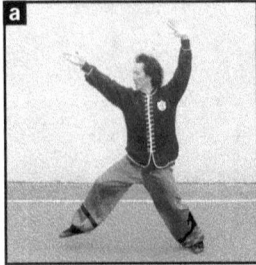

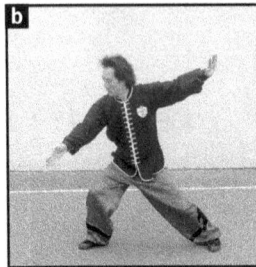

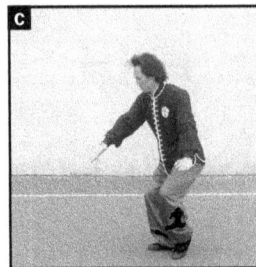

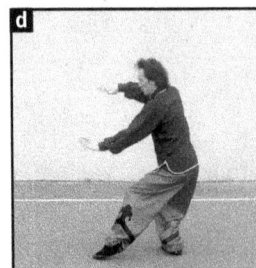

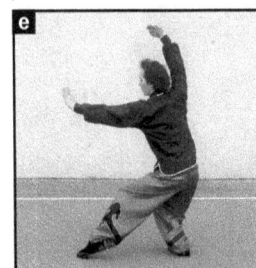

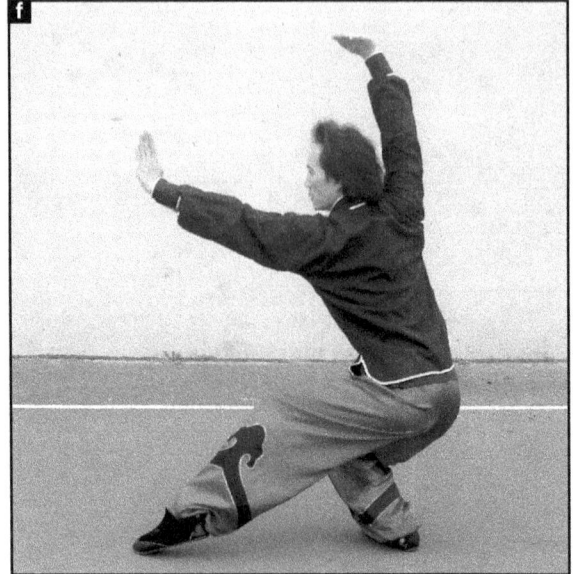

十、　上步撩陰掌

11 - Step forward. Uppercut palm strike to the groin.

As you stamp the ground with your right foot and step forward with the left leg into a left cat stance, make a counter-clockwise circular motion with the right hand, and strike upward with the fingertips of the left hand. The right hand moves from right to left, then down, and then upward.

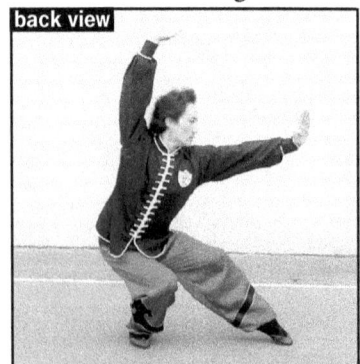

back view

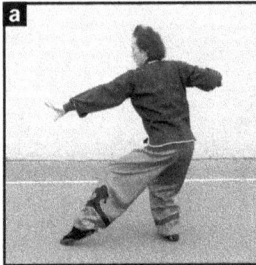

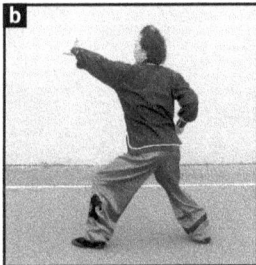

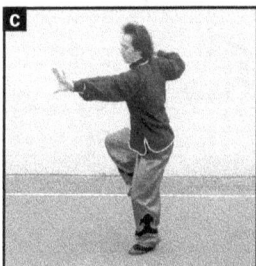

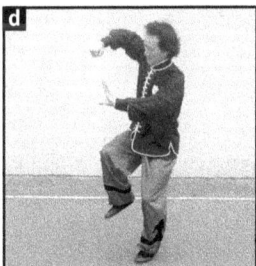

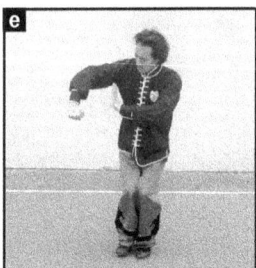

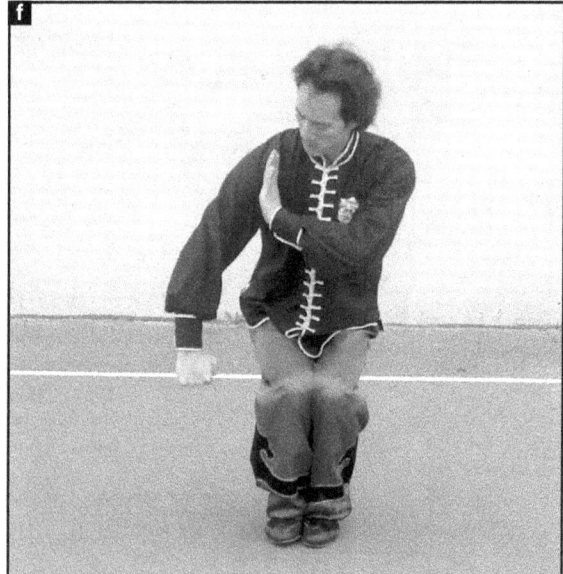

十三、 恨 地 栽 錘

12 - Stamp the ground. Strike with the fist.

Shift the weight onto the left foot, raise the right foot and then stamp the right foot down, ending alongside the left foot. The left hand will make a counter-clockwise circular clearing motion, followed by the downward punch of the right hand.

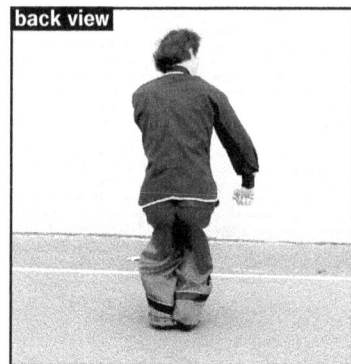

back view

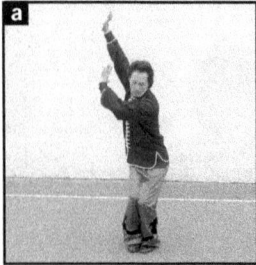

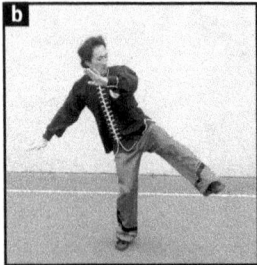

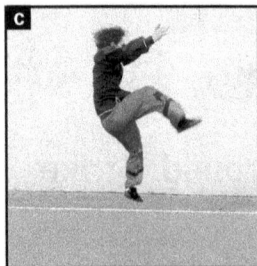

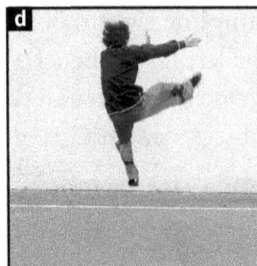

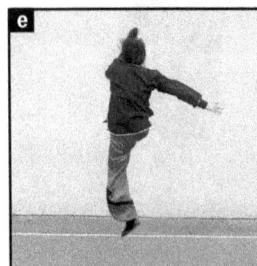

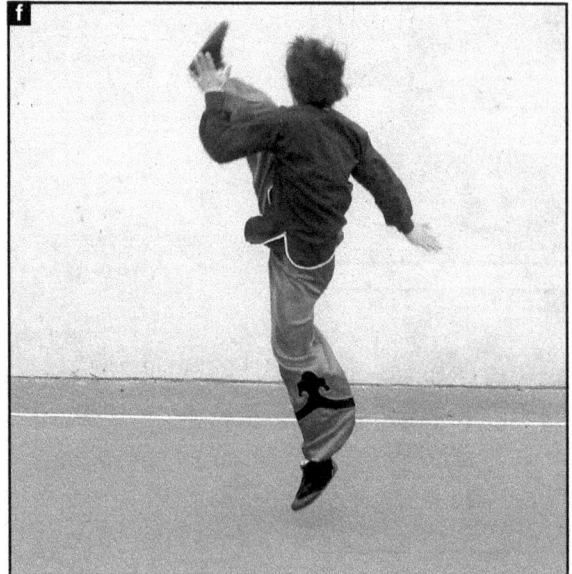

十三、 旋風腿

13 - Tornado kick.

Lift the left leg, and push off strongly with the right leg. The left leg will trace a counter-clockwise circle in the air, followed by the right leg. Use the left palm to slap the inside of the right foot.

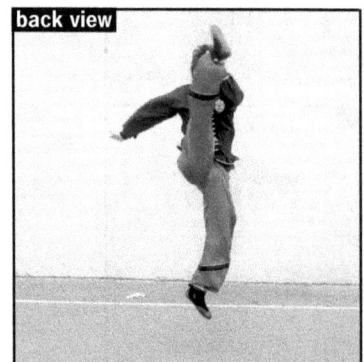

back view

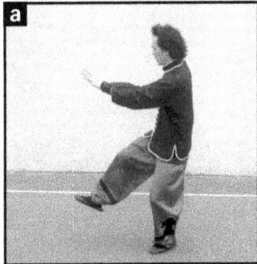

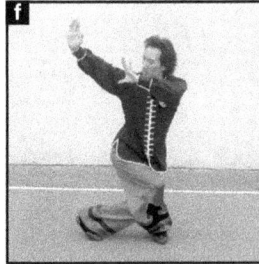

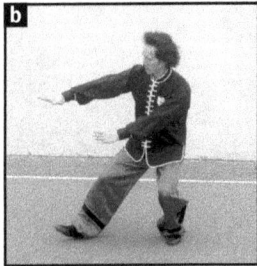

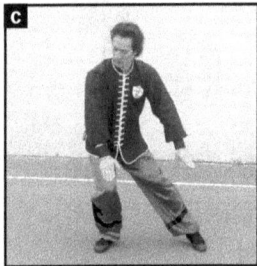

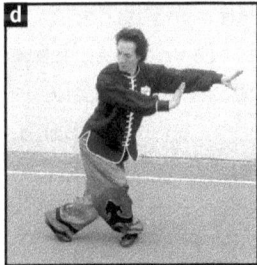

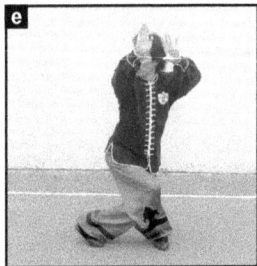

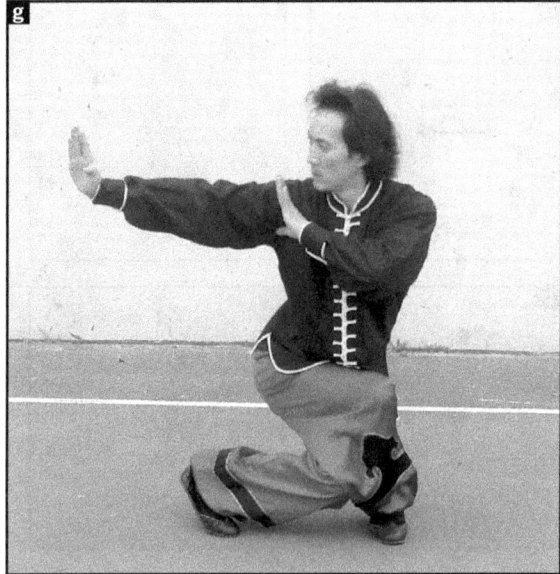

十四，偷步仙女散花

14 - Goddess sprinkles the flowers.

As your right foot steps down and forward, swing both arms in a clockwise circle together. As the left foot steps behind the right leg and forward into the right T-stance, bring both arms down together, the right edge of the palm facing ahead, and the left palm in the "guard" position against the inside of the right shoulder.

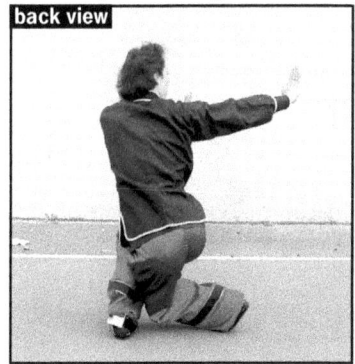

back view

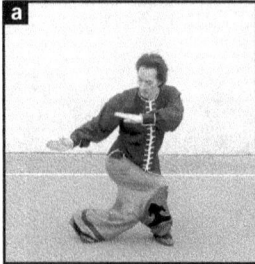

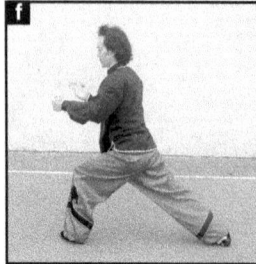

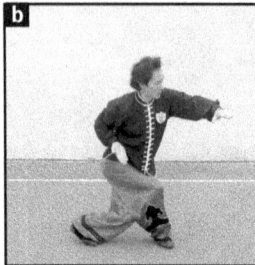

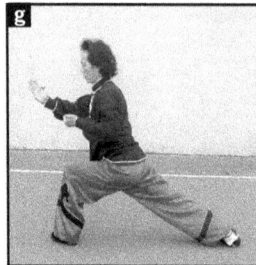

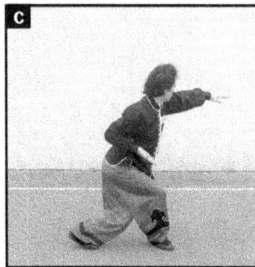

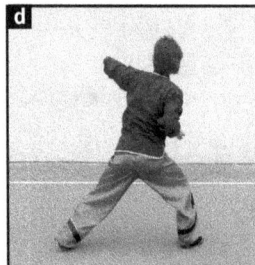

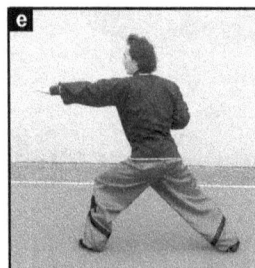

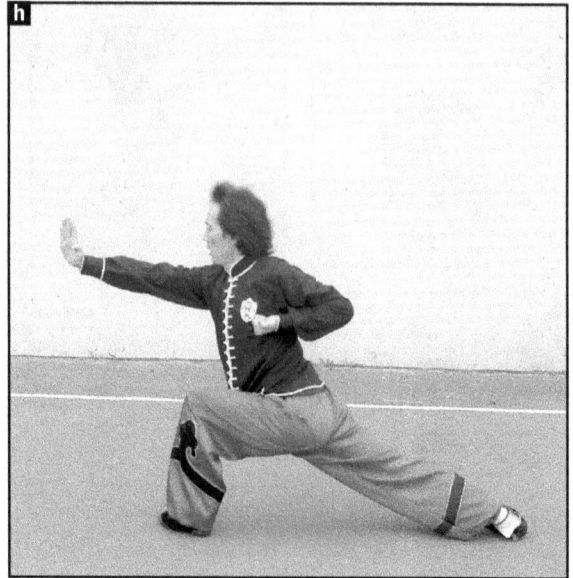

十五． 青 龍 轉 身

15A - Green dragon turns the body. (Right palm strike).

Turn your body to the left and make a clearing motion with the left open hand. As you shift into a left bow stance and your left hand withdraws to your side as a fist, strike straight with the blade edge of the right palm.

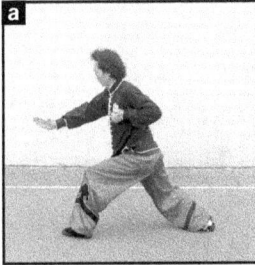

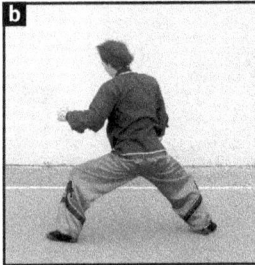

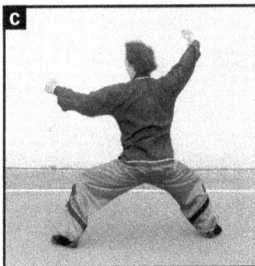

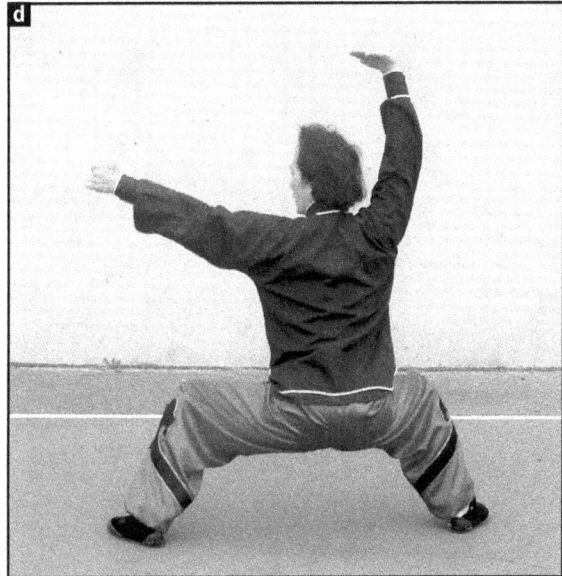

十五. 坐 馬 架 打 式

15B - Sit in a horse stance. Block and strike. (Left fist).

Then withdraw the right hand using an upward arcing clockwise motion. While blocking upward with the right hand and shifting into a horse stance, strike with a left vertical fist.

Alternatively, you may withdraw the right hand in a downward arcing motion and then moving it in a counterclockwise path until it stops at a position above your head.

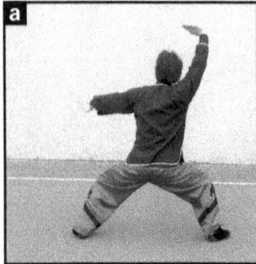

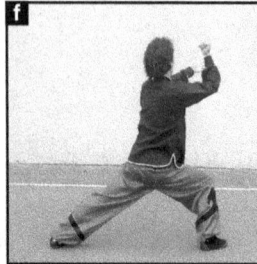

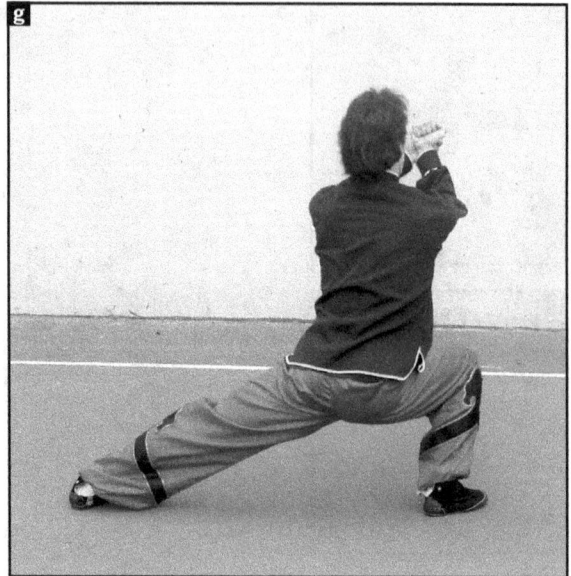

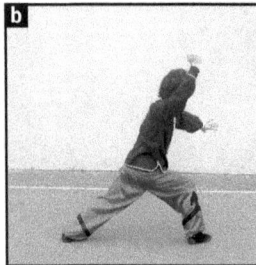

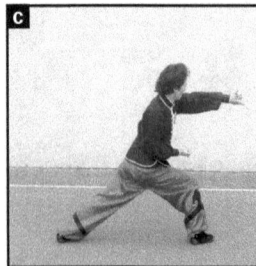

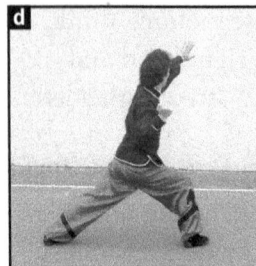

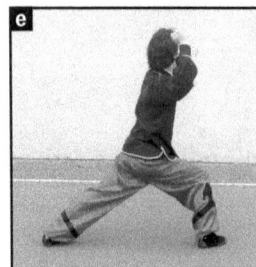

十六, 泰山壓頂右弓式

16 - Tai Mountain collapses on the head. Right bow stance.

Turn your body slightly to the right and make a large counter-clockwise clearing motion with the left hand. The right hand will mimic this motion of the left hand because the right hand will also make a counter-clockwise circle as it rises up as a fist to strike into the left palm. Shift into a right bow stance.

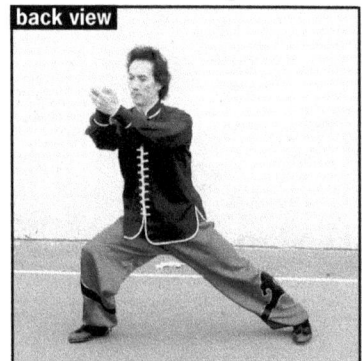

back view

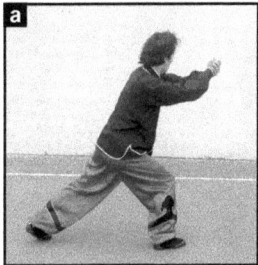

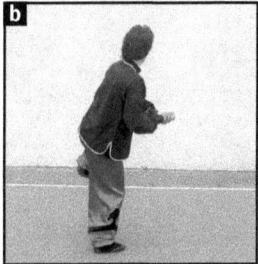

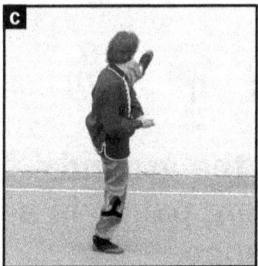

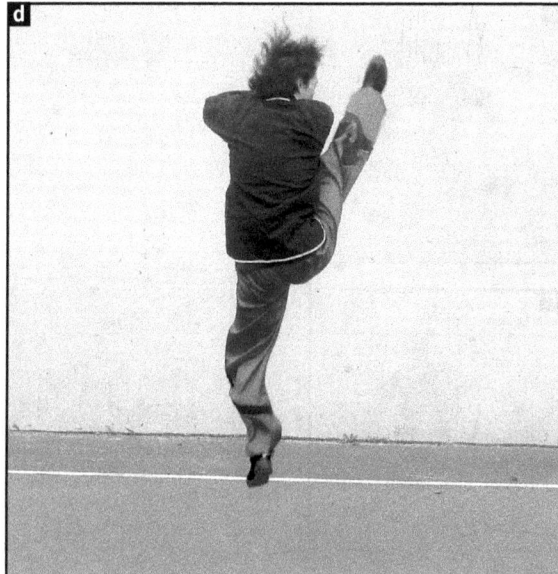

十七、落地雙推拳

17A - Continuous flying kick.

Kick up with the left leg, and your hands will move to your right side. Then move your hands to your left side as you do a double kick and use your right leg to strike with power.

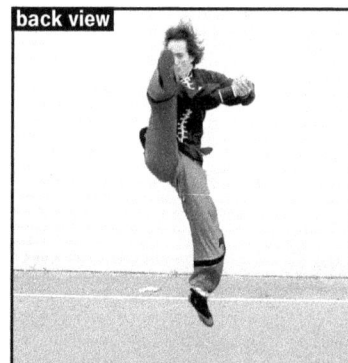

back view

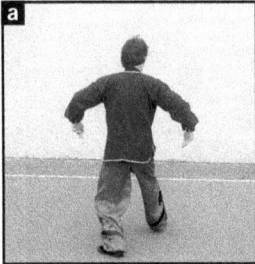

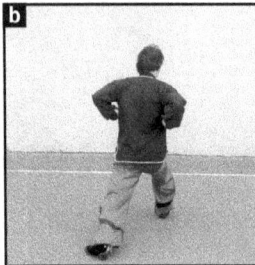

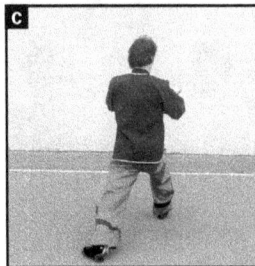

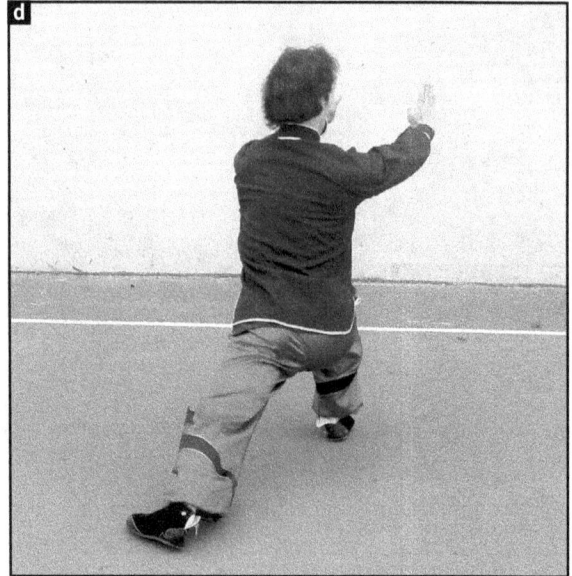

十七、連環飛踢

17B - Fall down to the ground. Double pushing palms in a right bow stance.

Fall forward into a right bow stance and push forward with both palms using the blade edge.

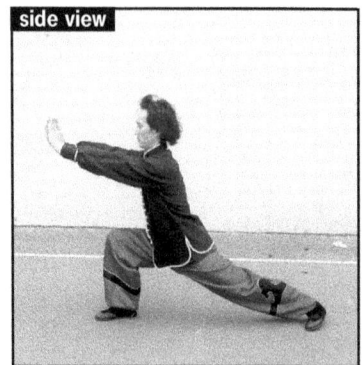
side view

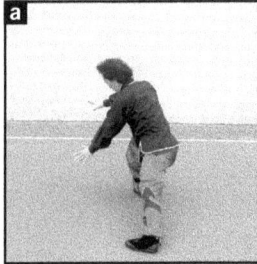

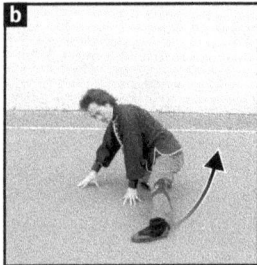

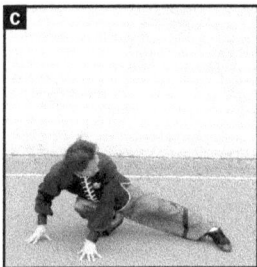

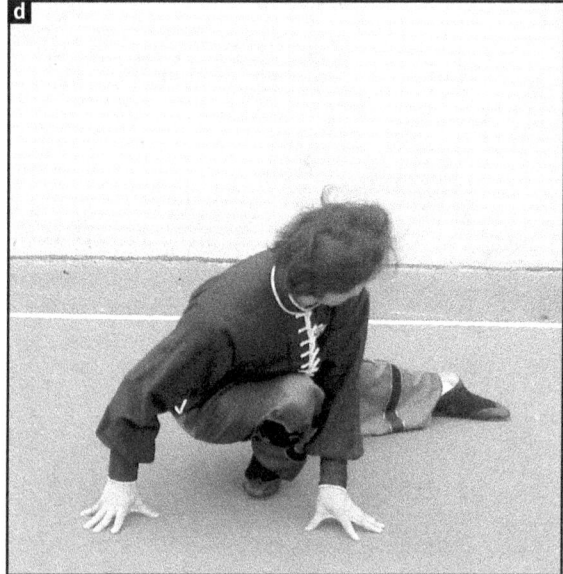

十八、後掃堂

18A - Back sweep.

Turn to your left; put both hands on the floor and do a left leg back sweep.

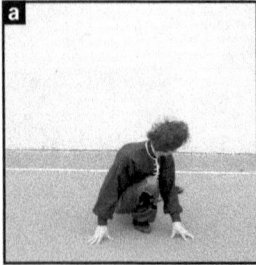

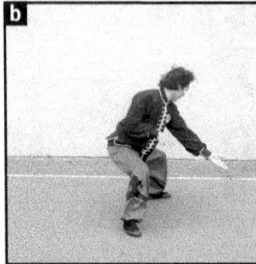

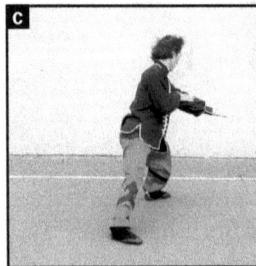

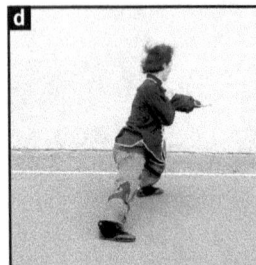

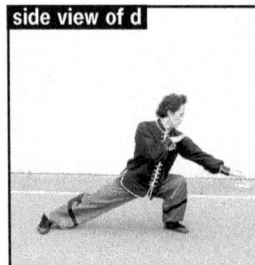

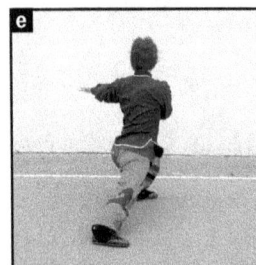

十八、鷹子抓肩

18B - Hawk grabs the shoulder. (Right palm strike).

As you shift into a left bow stance, place your right hand (palm down) against the left side of your chest. Open your left hand and swing your left arm in a large clockwise circle, first forward, and then back.

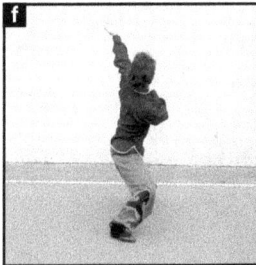

f

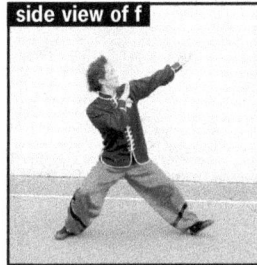

side view of f

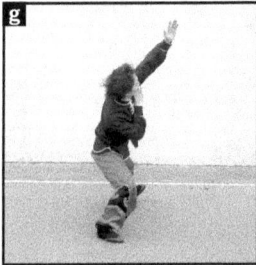

g

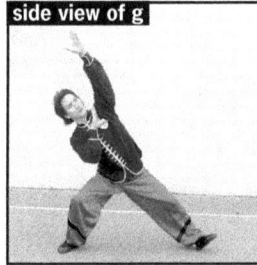

side view of g

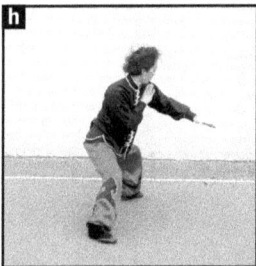

h

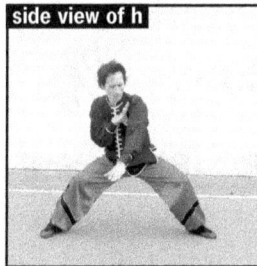

side view of h

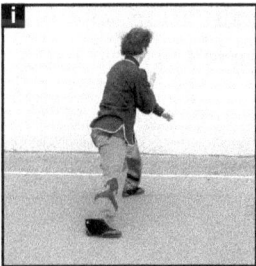

i

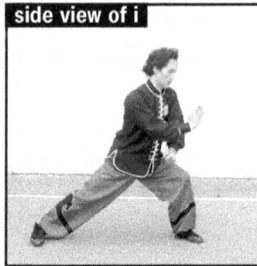

side view of i

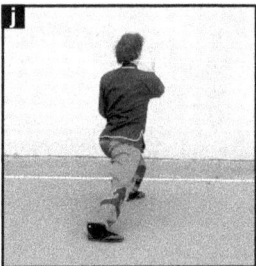

j

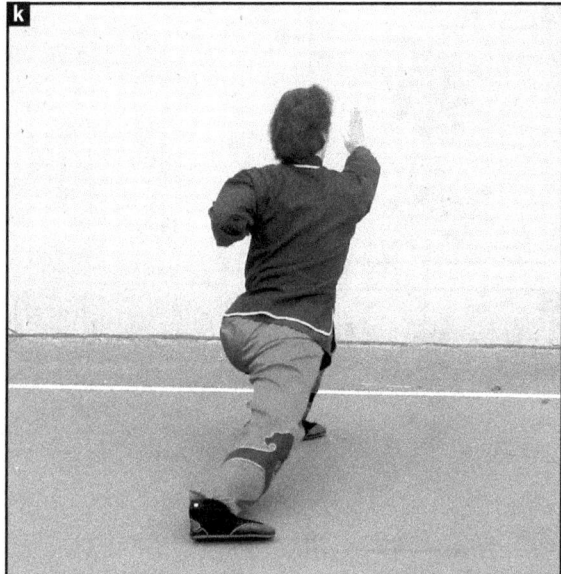

k

十八、鷹 子 抓 肩

18B - Continued.

When the left arm comes back, shift the weight to the right (back) leg, and only the left heel will be on the ground. (**a** to **g**)

Then fall forward and shift back into the left bow stance, as your left hand makes a downward clearing motion and withdraws into a fist at your left side, while the right arm pushes out into a strike using the blade edge of the right palm. (**h** to **k**)

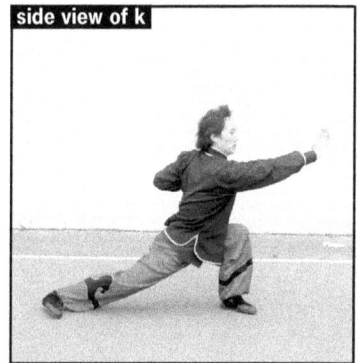

side view of k

45

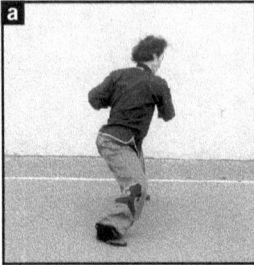

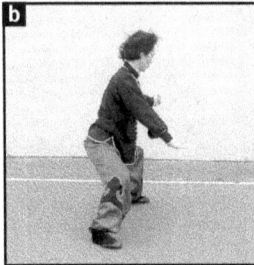

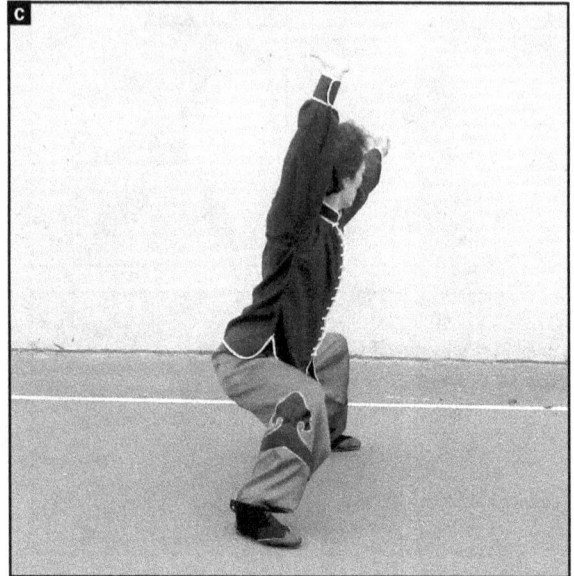

十八、 架 打 式

18C -Block and strike. (Left fist strike).

Withdraw the right hand and block upward. The right palm ends facing upward. The left hand strikes with a left vertical fist.

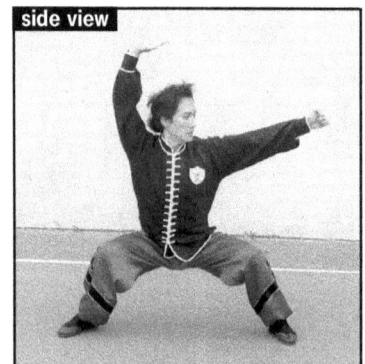

side view

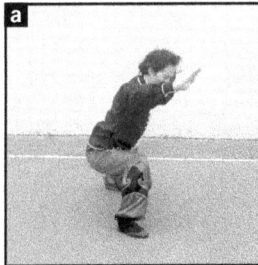

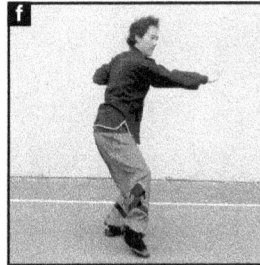

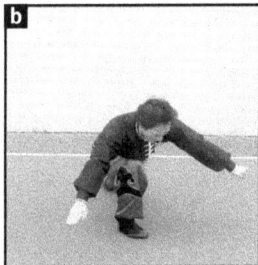

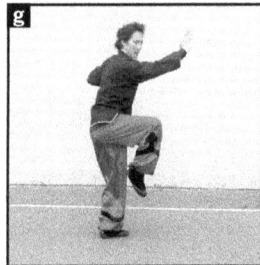

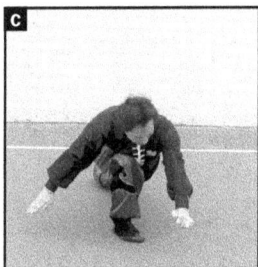

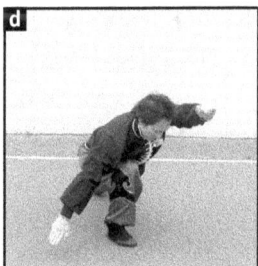

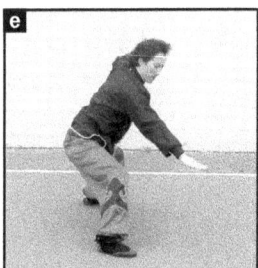

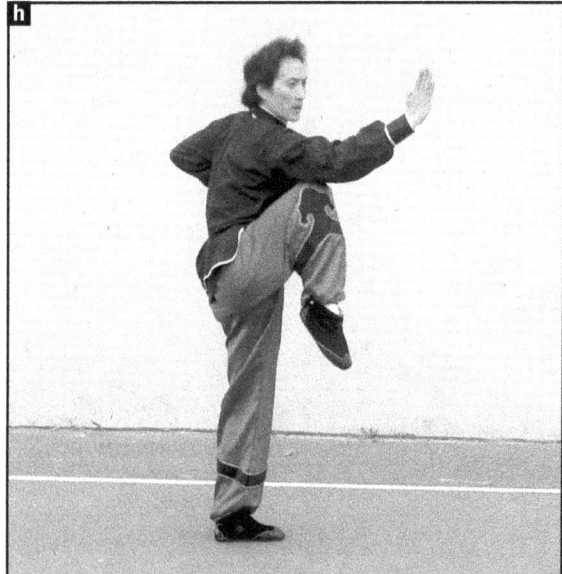

十九、左 右 撐 手 獨 立 勢

19 - Left and right, flip the hands upward. Crane stance (single leg).

Then turn toward your right side, and bend down onto your right leg and swing your right arm in a large clockwise circle. As the right arm moves in a clockwise motion, the left arm will make a counter-clockwise circle. As you rise back up onto the left leg into a crane stance, the left fist will withdraw to the waist as the right palm comes to the front of your face. Your right leg is raised up and you look past your right hand.

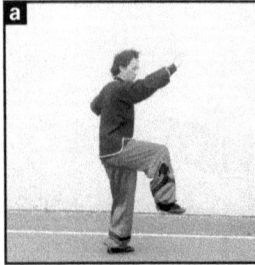

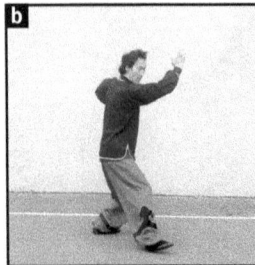

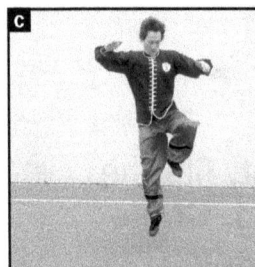

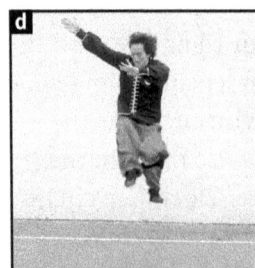

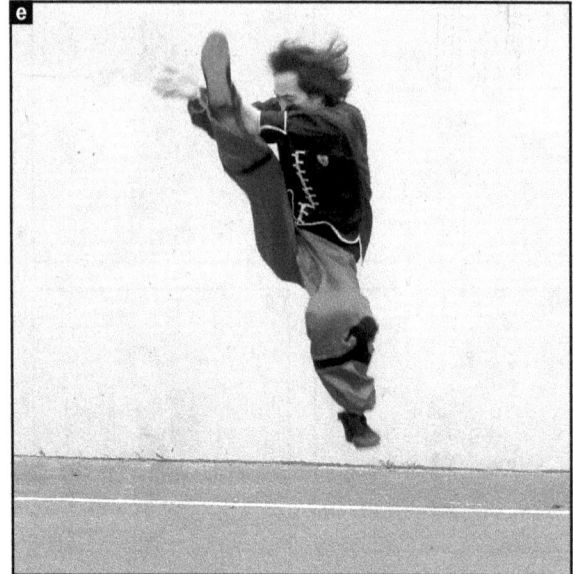

二十、轉 身 右 擺 蓮 腿

20 - Turn around. Right leg flying lotus kick.

Step down with the right leg and then push off hard with the right foot as you rotate your body in a clockwise motion. The left leg will swing up, followed by the large, clockwise swinging motion of the right leg. You are in the air! Slap the instep of the right foot with first the left palm, followed by the right palm. As you strike your right foot with your hands your fingers will point to your right. Your body will revolve in a complete circle in the air.

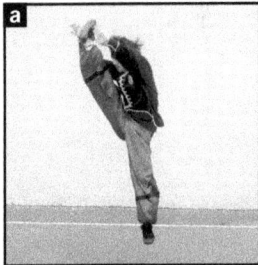

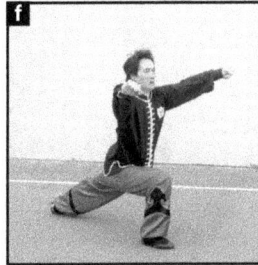

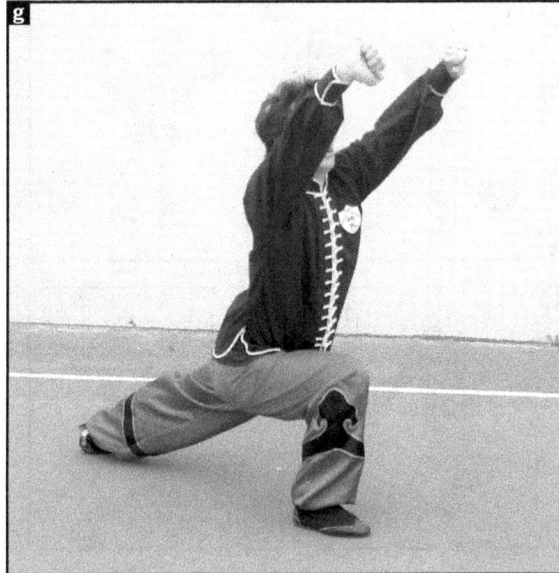

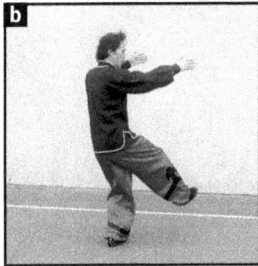

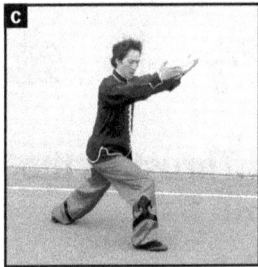

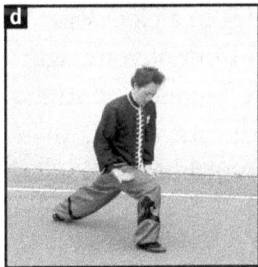

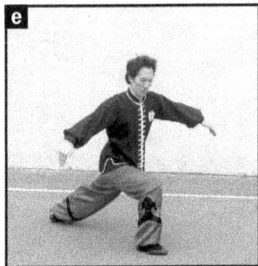

二一、落地雙風貫耳拳

21 - Come down to the ground. Double wind strikes the ears. Right bow stance.

Your left leg will land first, followed by the right leg. As you continue to turn to your right, begin to shift into a right bow stance. As you are starting to rise up, brush the backs of both hands against the top of your thighs. Then strike forward with the knuckles of the backs of both of your hands. You will end in a right bow stance.

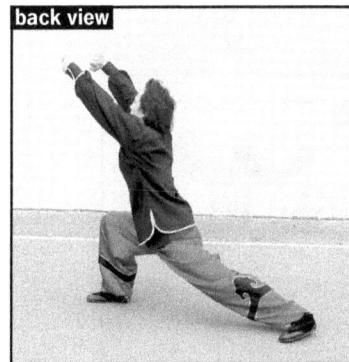

back view

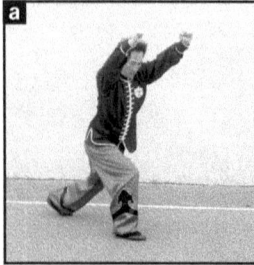

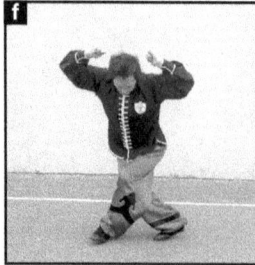

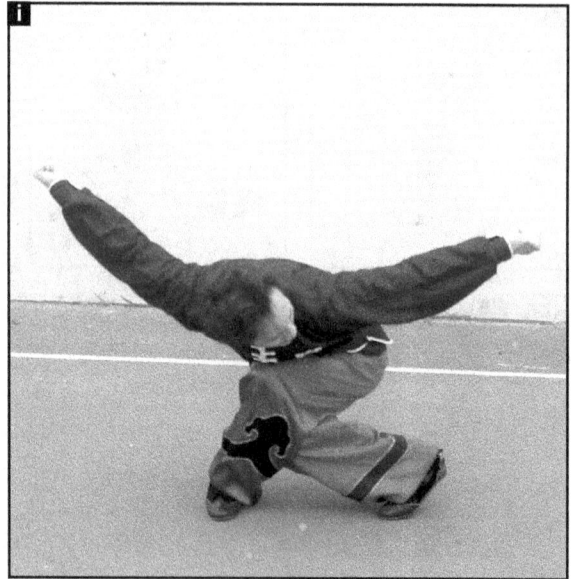

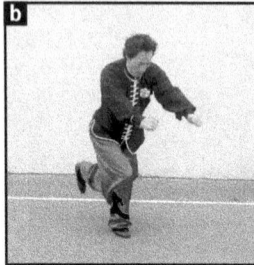

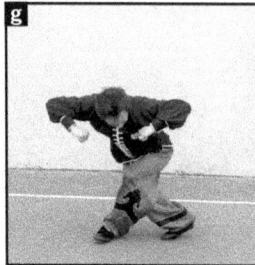

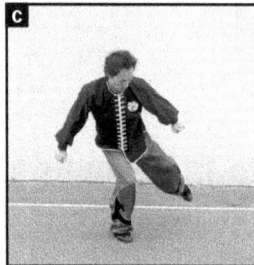

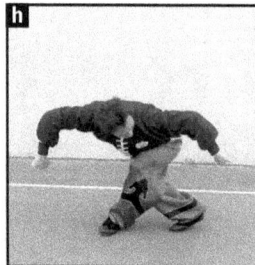

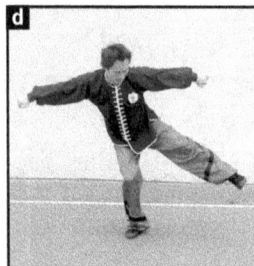

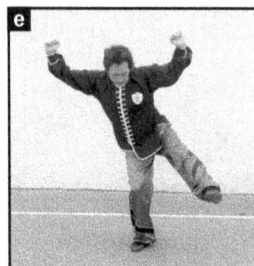

二二・拗步分插錘

22 - Twist stance. Thrust to the groin with both fists.

While swinging both fists down, lift the left leg and move the left leg in a clockwise motion so that it passes in front of your right leg. As you shift into a left T-stance, continue the circular motion of both fists, up and then down, to finally strike outward on both sides. Look to your left.

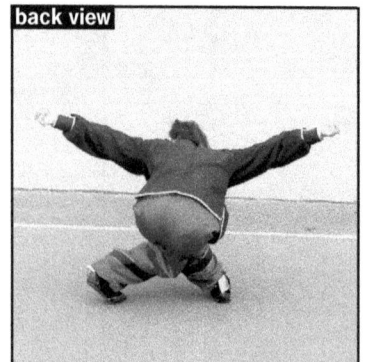

back view

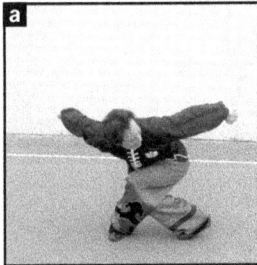

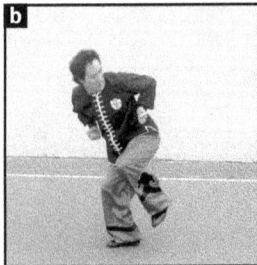

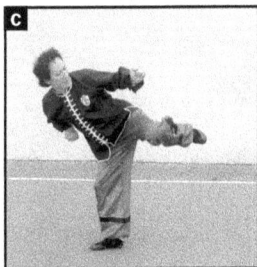

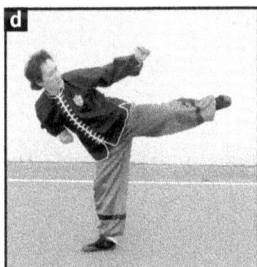

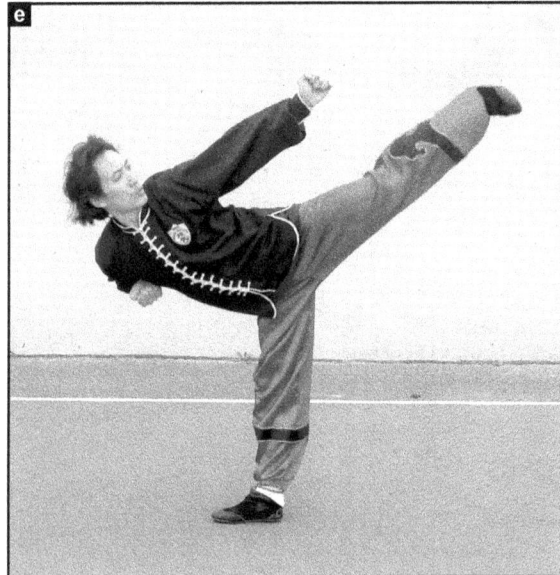

二三、挑手左蹬

23A - Flipping hand (fist), left thrust kick.

Lift the left leg and do a left side kick while the left fist punches out at the same time.

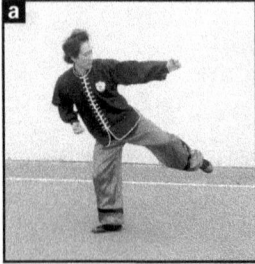

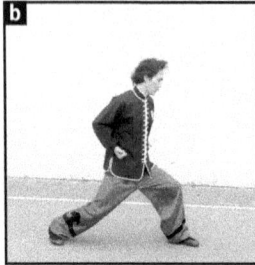

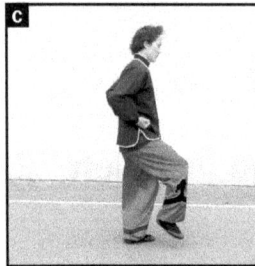

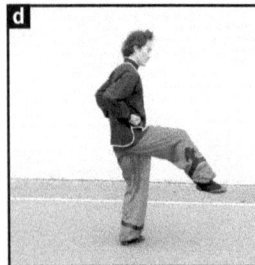

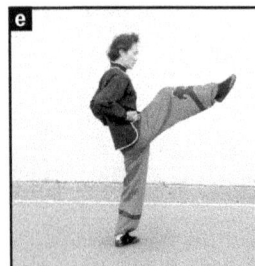

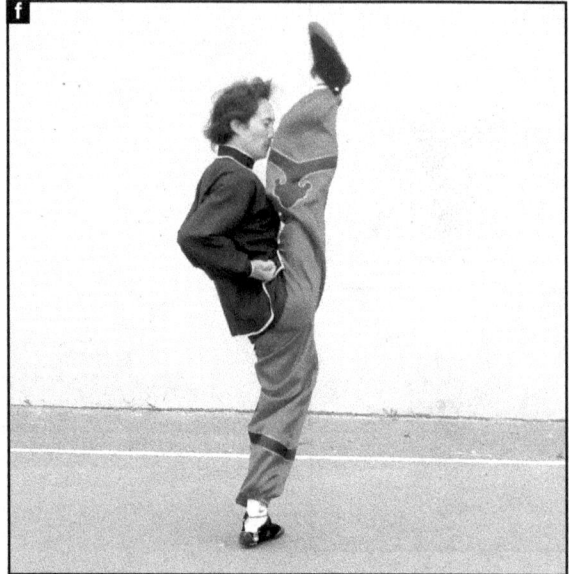

二三、右踢

23B - Right toe kick.

Step down with the left leg; bring both fists to the sides of your waist and do a high right leg toe kick.

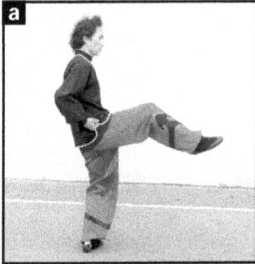

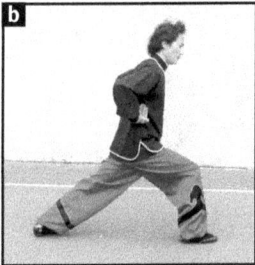

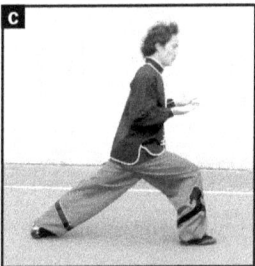

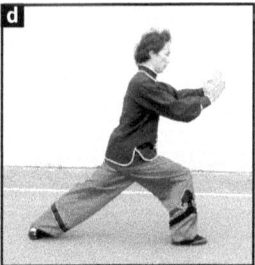

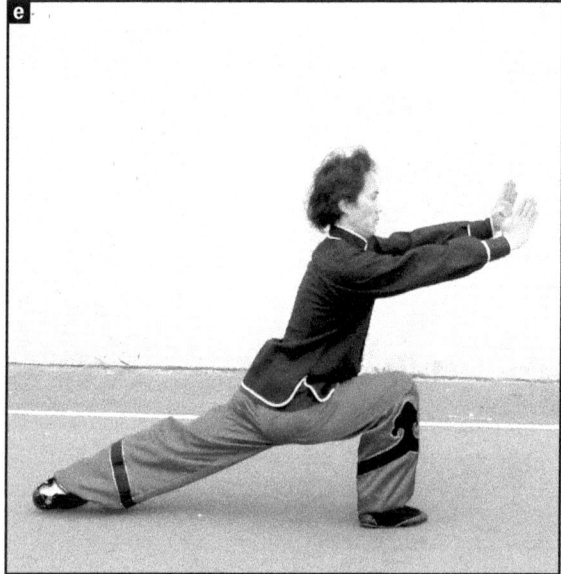

二三、雙推掌

23C - Double pushing palm.

Step down with the right leg into a right bow stance. As you shift into the right bow stance, push out with the blade edge of both palms.

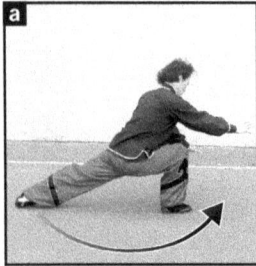

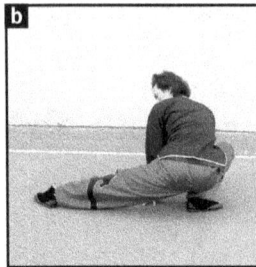

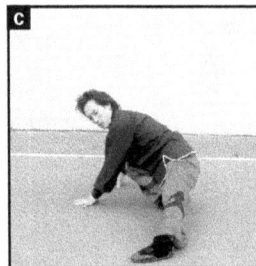

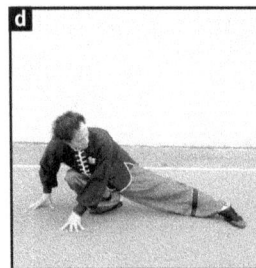

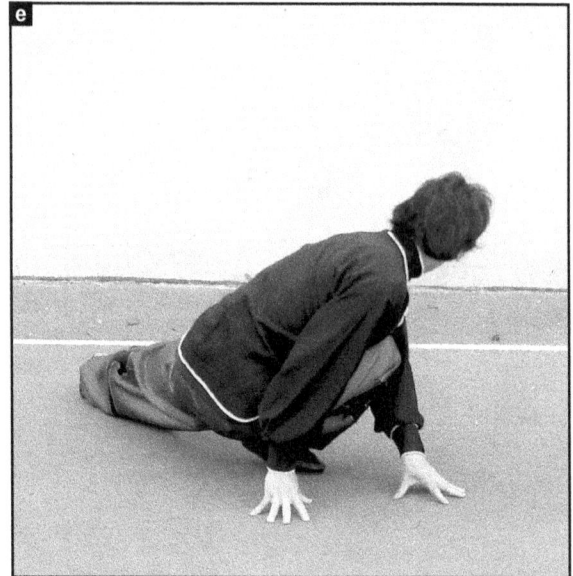

二四、後掃堂腿

24 - Full back sweep.

Turn towards your left and place both hands on the ground. Do a complete left leg back sweep.

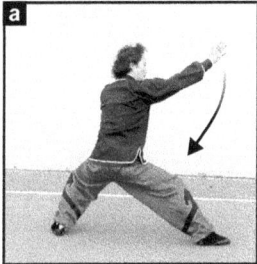

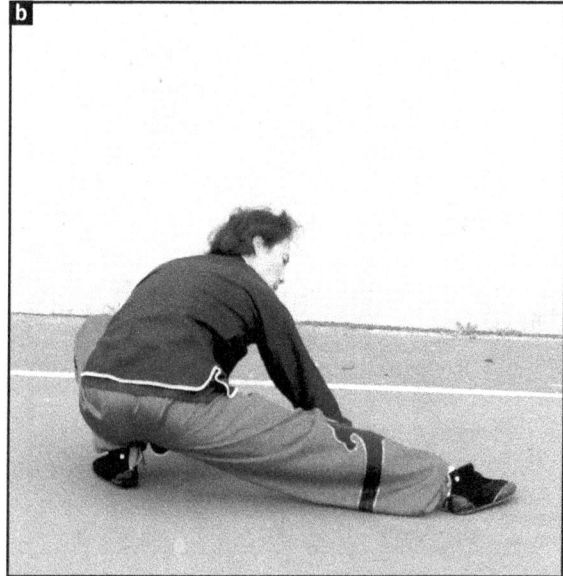

二五、拍地飛沙

25 - Slap the ground. Flying sand.

As you finish your turn, rise up slightly and then slap the ground hard as you end in a right scattered stance.

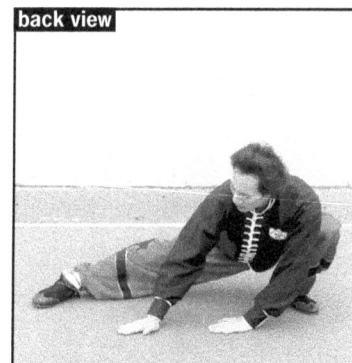

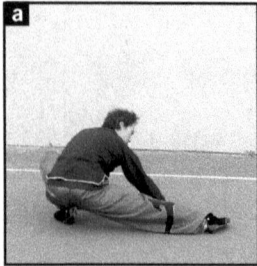

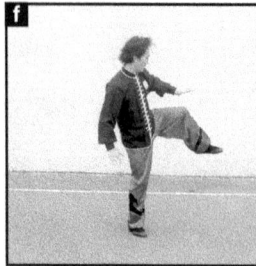

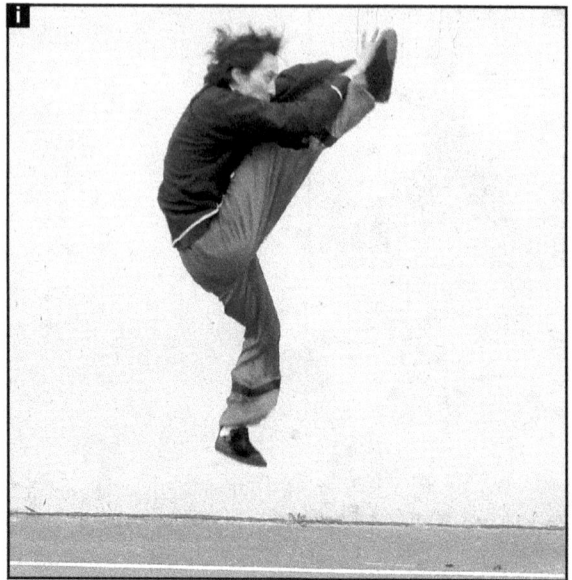

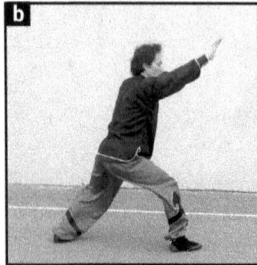

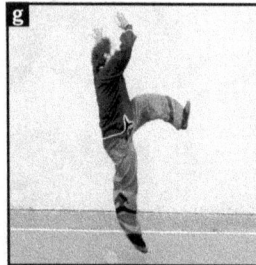

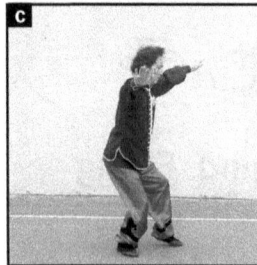

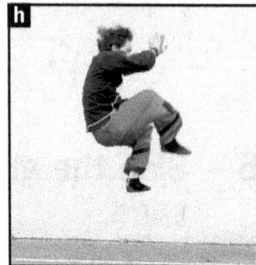

二六、二起腿

26 - Double kick.

Rise up, run forward and do a double kick with the right leg, slapping the instep of the right foot with the right hand.

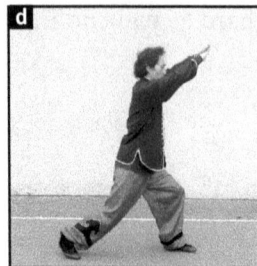

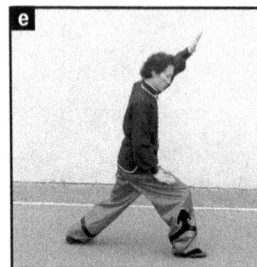

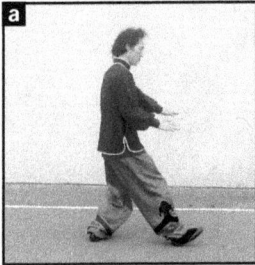

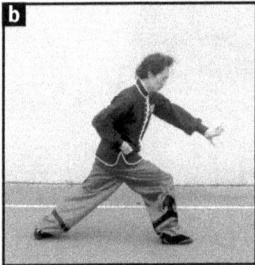

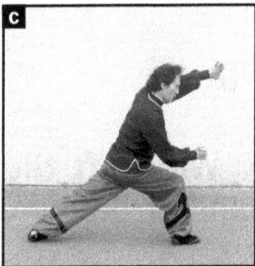

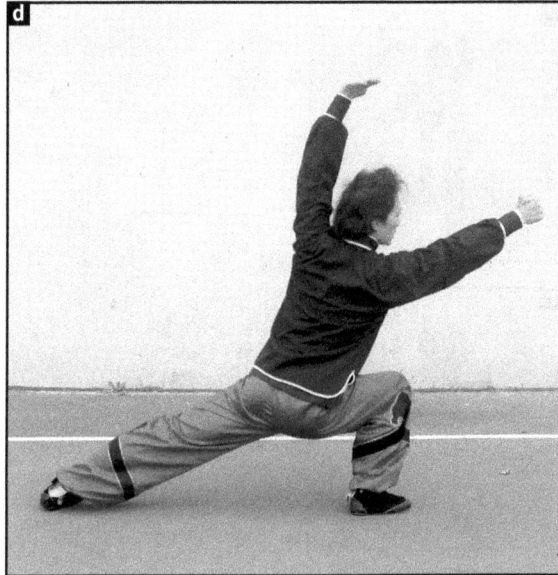

二七，落地弓步架打式

27 - Come down to the ground. Right bow stance. Block and strike. (Left blocks and right fist strikes).

As you fall into a right bow stance, block upward with the left hand and strike forward with a right vertical fist.

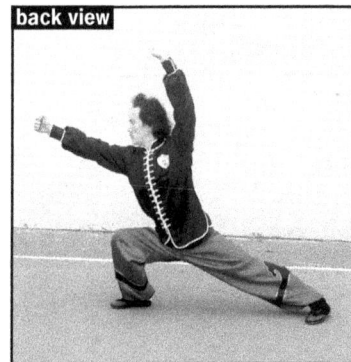

back view

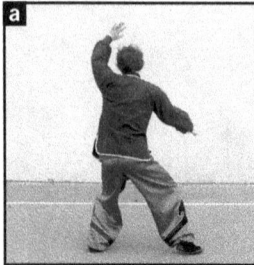

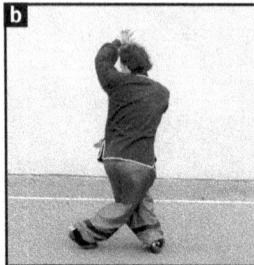

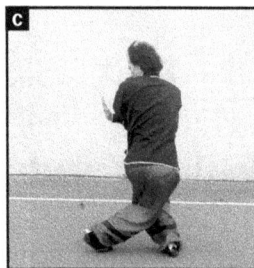

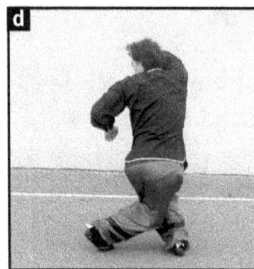

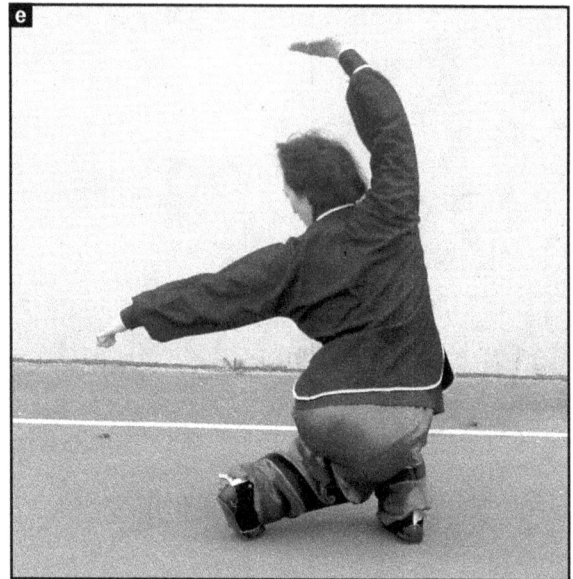

二八、偷步脱手架打式

28 - Steal a step. Wipe off the hand. Block and strike.

Then step the right foot back in the opposite direction, past the back of the left leg, into a left T-stance. As the right foot steps back, the right hand will drop down and then up, using a large clockwise motion. The left horizontal fist, staying inside the motion of the open right hand, will make a clockwise downward motion to finally strike back and downward as the right hand rises up.

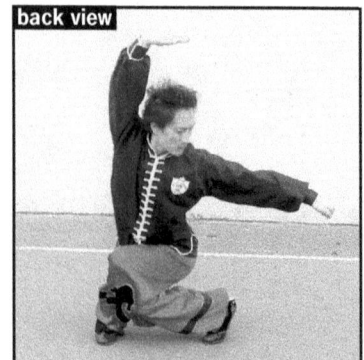

back view

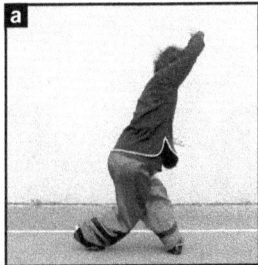

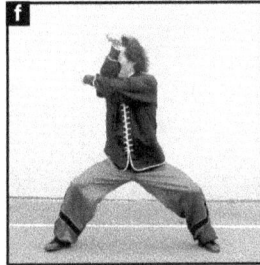

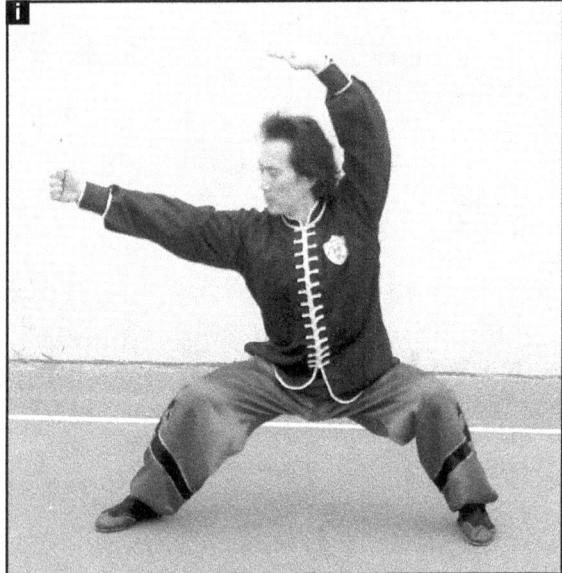

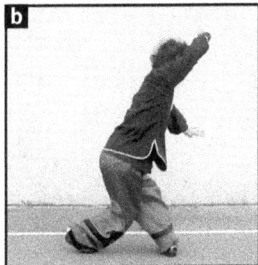

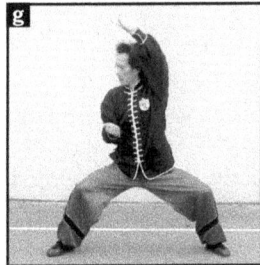

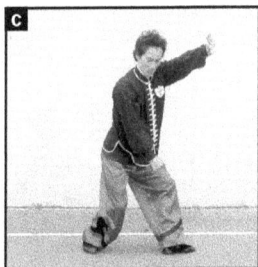

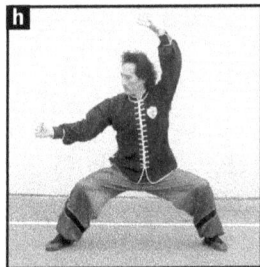

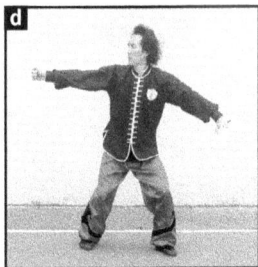

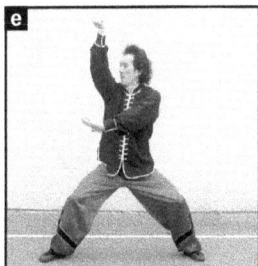

二九、轉 身 坐 馬 架 打 式

29 - Turn around. Sit in a horse stance. Block and strike.

Turn your body to the right and all the way around. Sit in a horse stance. The right vertical fist will make a counter-clockwise motion and strike straight ahead. The right fist will stay on the inside as the left hand makes a counter-clockwise circle and blocks upward.

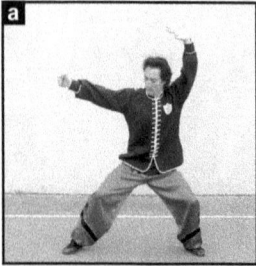

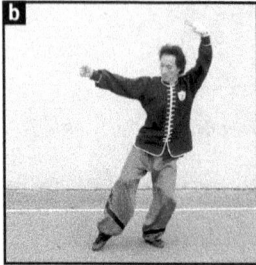

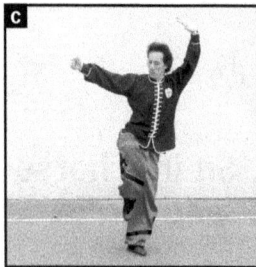

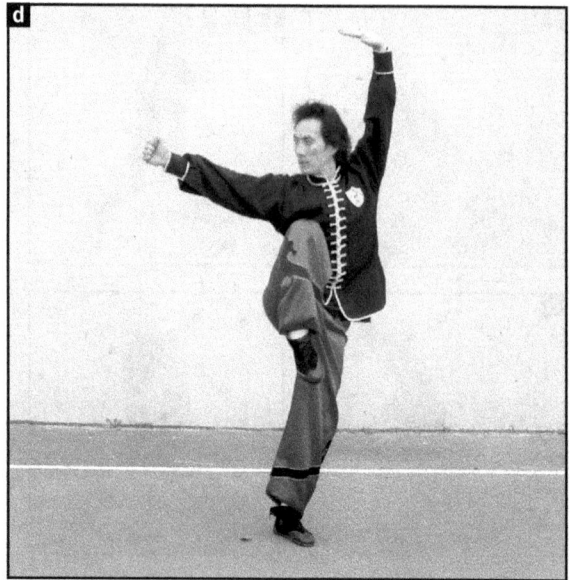

三十、震足

30A - Raise the right leg.

While you withdraw and raise the right leg, the weight shifts to your left leg as you move into a crane stance. The hand position does not change.

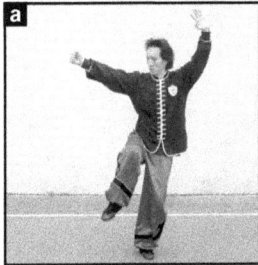

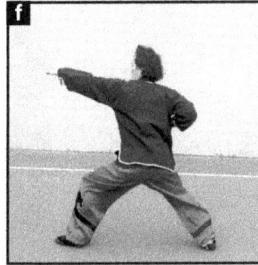

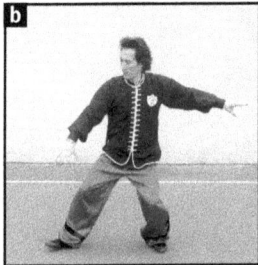

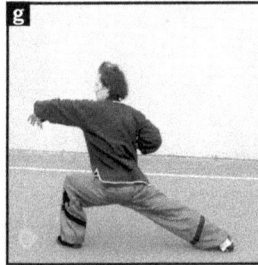

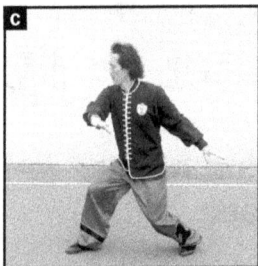

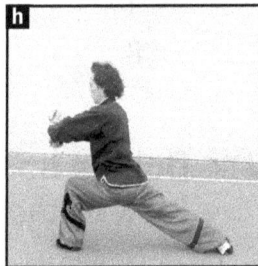

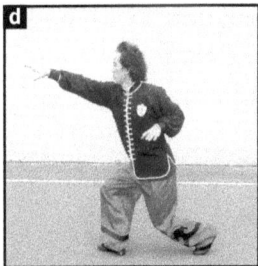

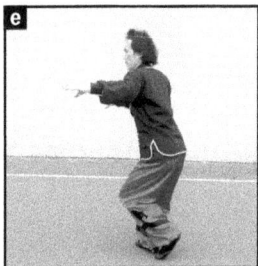

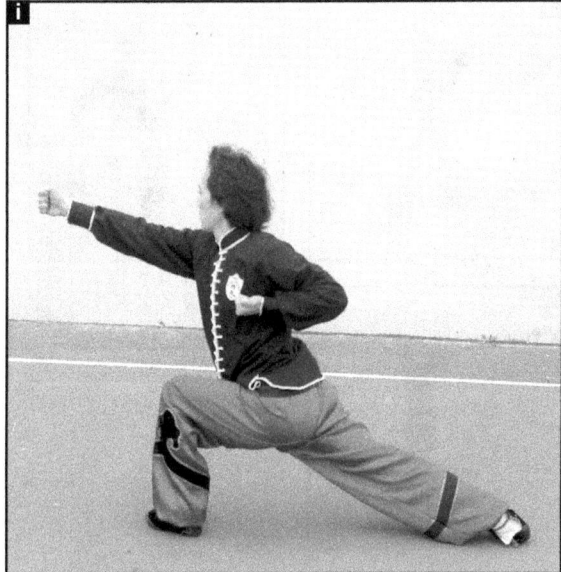

三十、震足纏手 上步壓打

30B -Stamp the foot. Tangling hand. Step forward. Press and strike with the fist.

Then, as you stamp your right foot on the ground, the right hand will make a clockwise circular grabbing motion, followed by a similar grabbing motion with the left hand. As the left hand withdraws to the side of the body as a fist, the right vertical fist strikes forward.

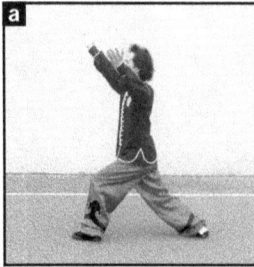

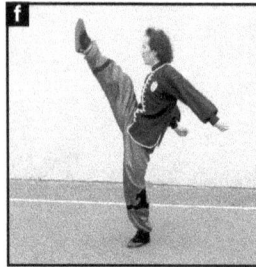

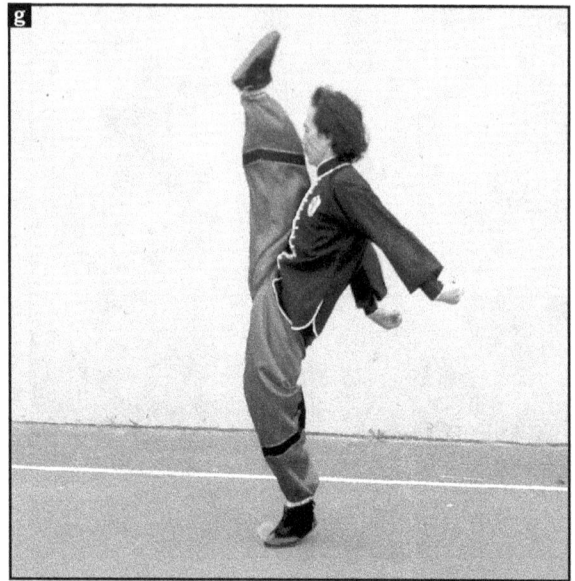

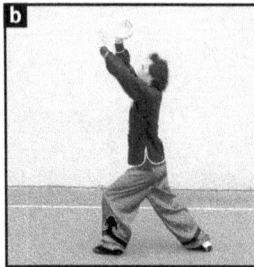

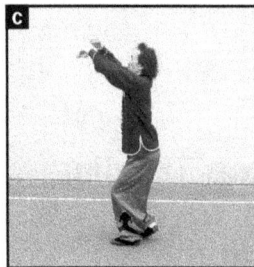

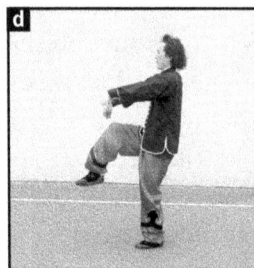

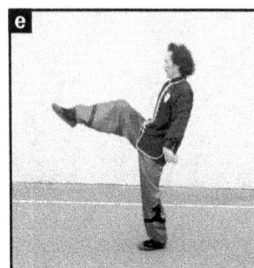

三一、雙鉤手迎面腿

31 - Double hooking hands. Kick to the face.

Open both hands as you raise them up in front of you. As you hook down with both hands using cranes' beaks, right forearm on top of the left, kick upward using a right leg toe kick.

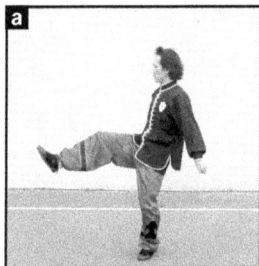

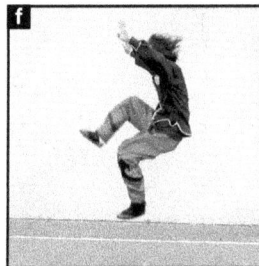

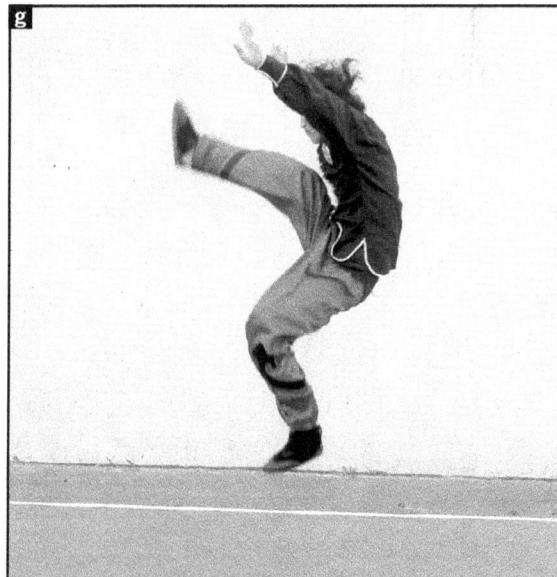

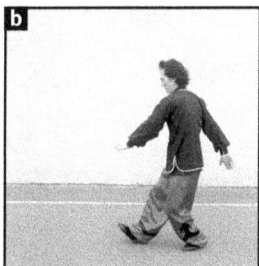

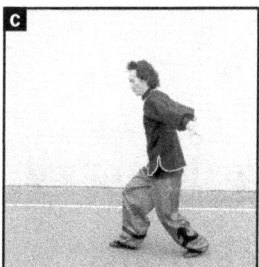

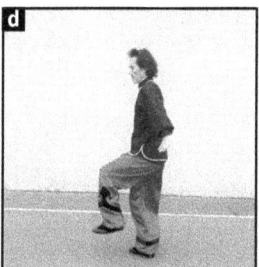

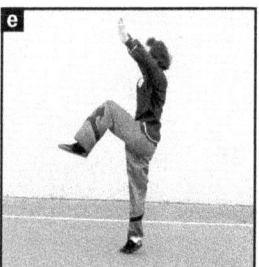

二二、雙捧飛踢

32A - Double uplifting hands. Flying kick.

Bring the right leg back down to the ground, and push off hard with the right leg as you swing the left leg up to begin the double kick. The back of the right hand will slap the inside of the left palm as both hands push up and outward as the right leg kicks up. A right flying heel kick is shown.

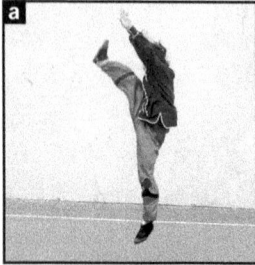

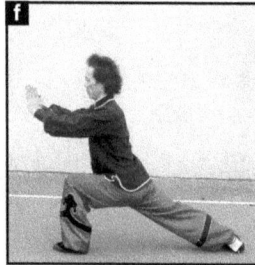

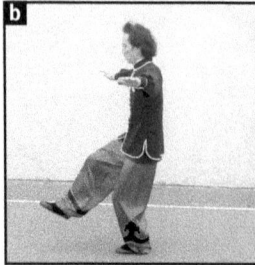

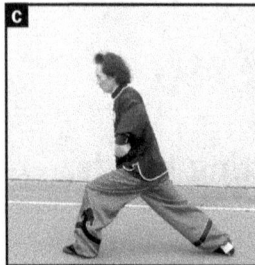

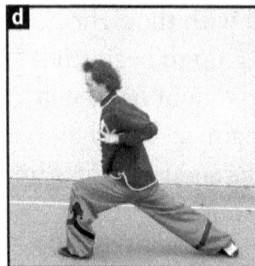

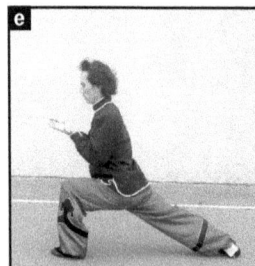

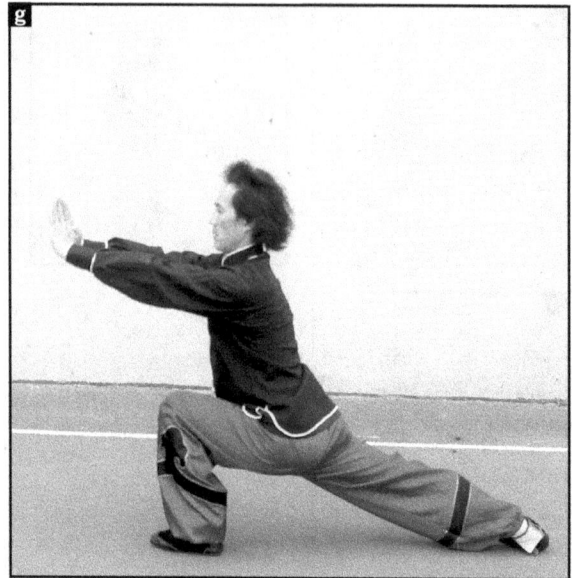

三二、落地退步雙推掌

32B -Come down to the ground in a left bow stance. Double pushing palms.

As you land on your left leg, withdraw your right leg and sit in a left bow stance. Both arms will push forward as you strike with the blade edge of both palms.

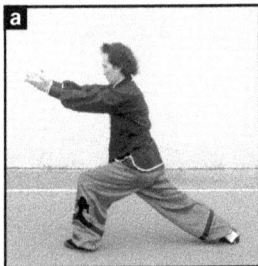

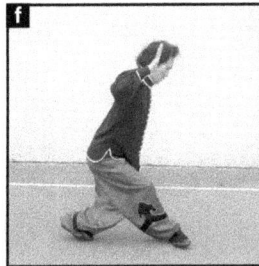

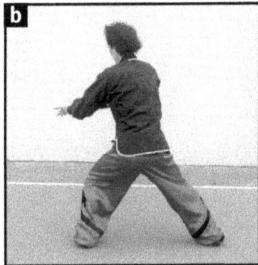

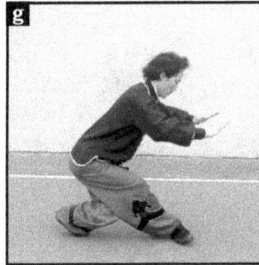

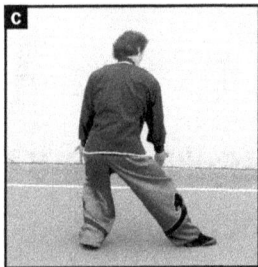

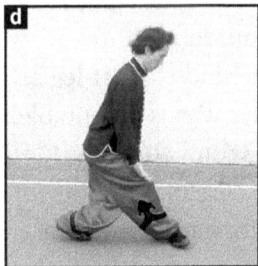

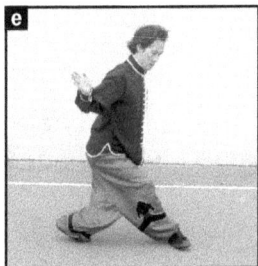

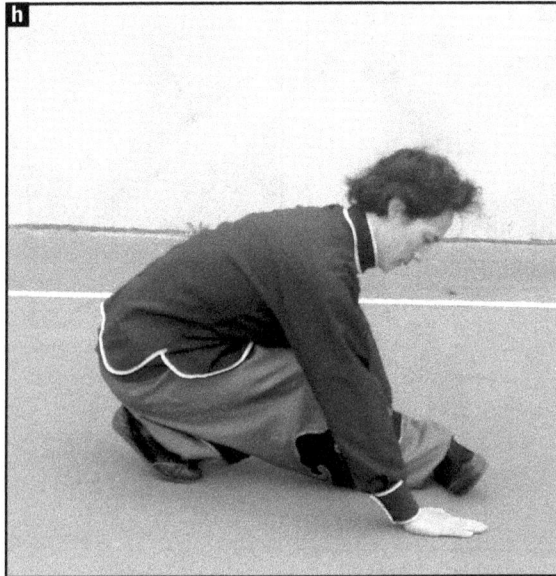

三三、回身坐盤拍地掌

33 - Turn around and slap the ground with the palms in a cross-legged stance.

Turn to your right, drop both hands downward and slap the top of both thighs with the back of both palms. Using circular motion, slap the ground with both palms as you sit on the floor in a right T-stance.

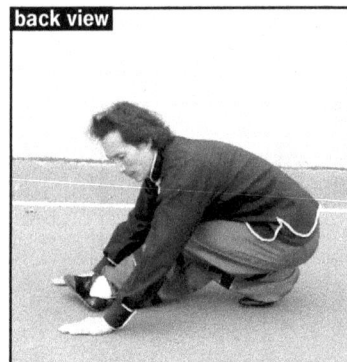

back view

65

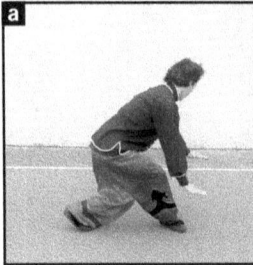

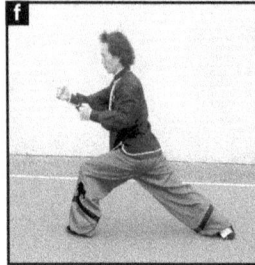

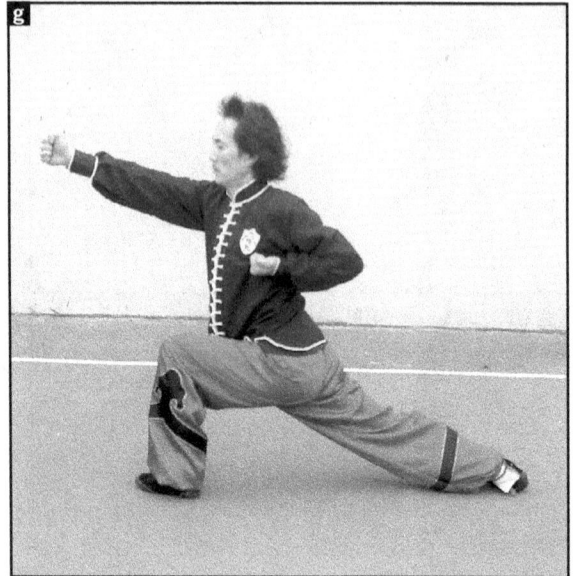

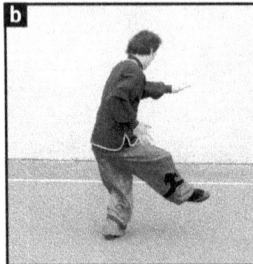

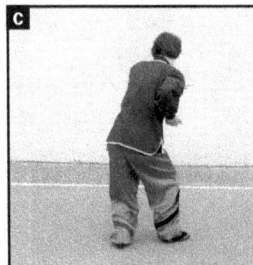

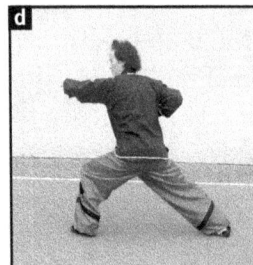

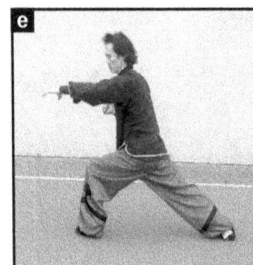

三四、 轉 身 摟 手 平 衡 拳

34 - Turn around. Pulling hand (Left). Straight punch (Right).

Turn to your left and lift your right foot off the ground and past your left leg. You may also step down just behind the left leg as shown in the photos. Either way is acceptable. As you stamp the ground with your right foot, make a counter-clockwise clearing motion with your left hand, step forward with your left leg into a left bow stance and strike with a right vertical fist.

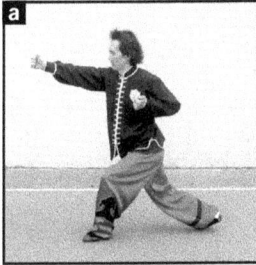

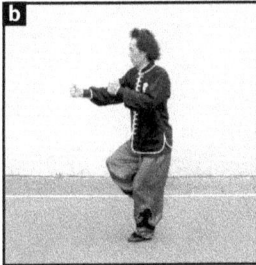

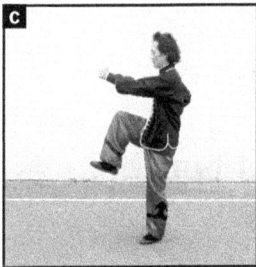

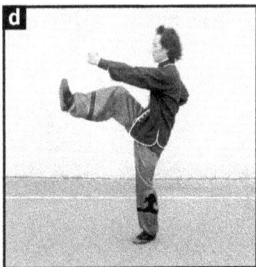

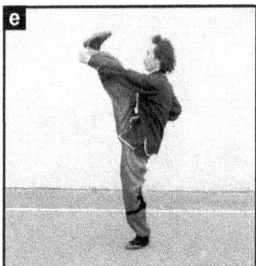

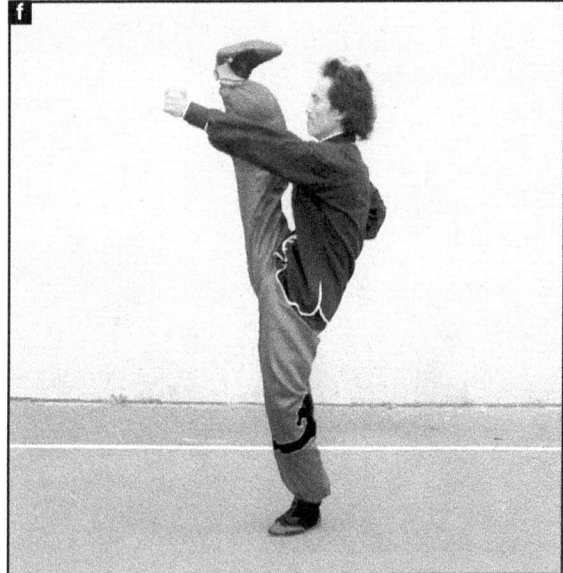

三五、右 踢 十 字 腿

35 - Right kick.

Turn your left foot slightly and strike with a left vertical fist while you perform a right leg heel kick.

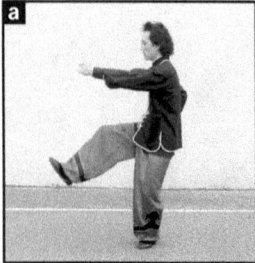

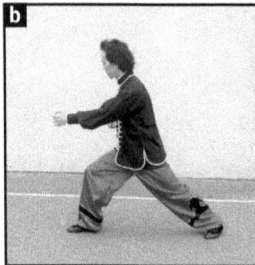

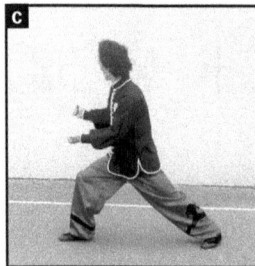

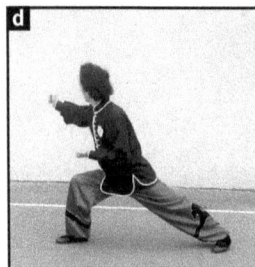

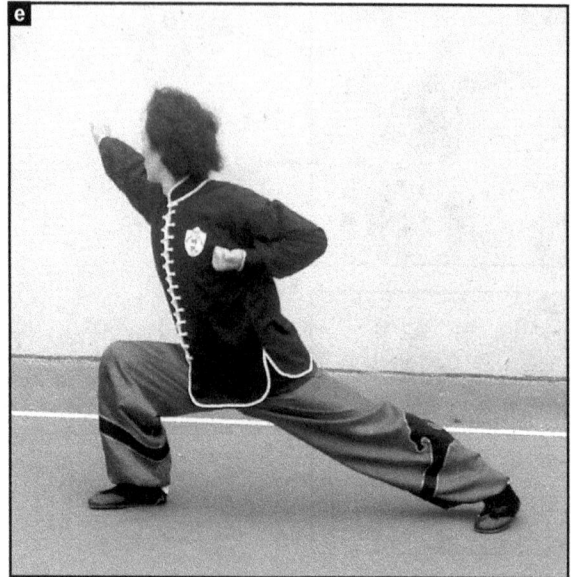

三六、右衝拳右弓式

36A -Right straight punch. Right bow stance

As you step down into a right bow stance, strike to your right side with a right vertical fist.

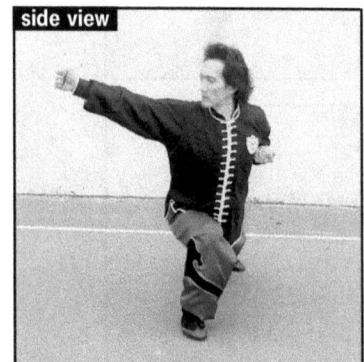

side view

68

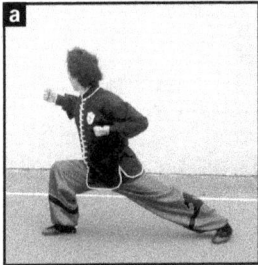

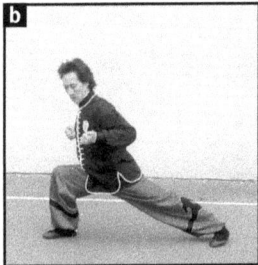

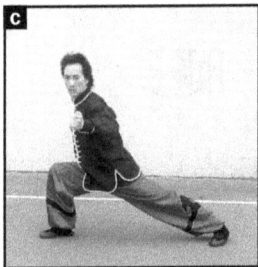

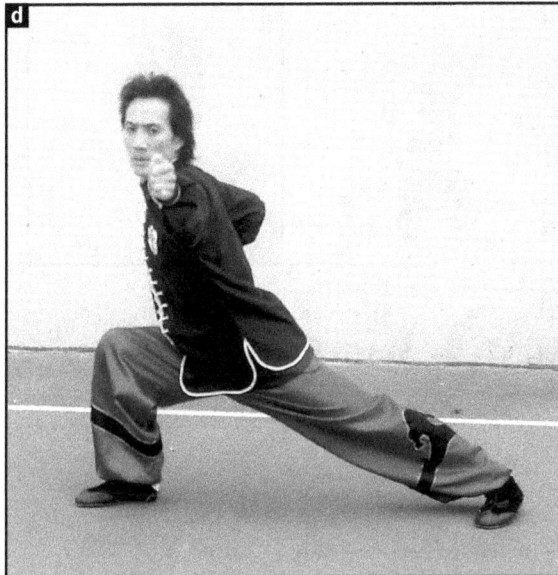

三六、 衝拳右弓式

36B -Left straight punch.
Right bow stance.

Then, look towards your left and strike out with a left vertical fist.

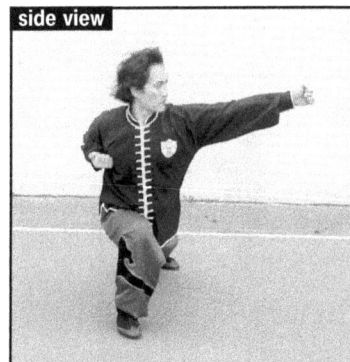

side view

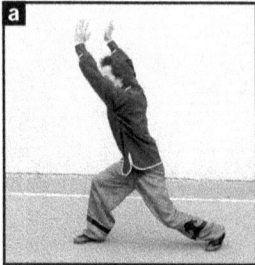

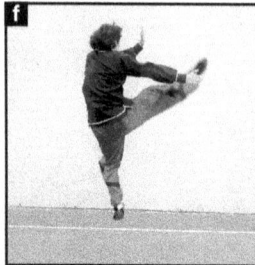

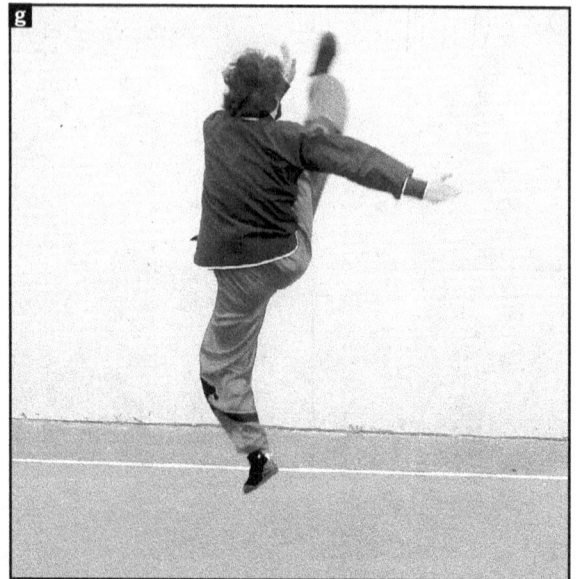

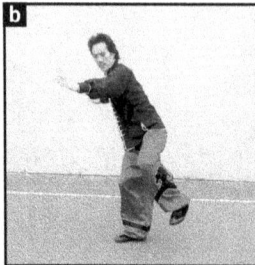

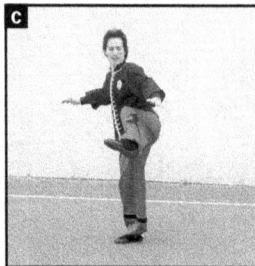

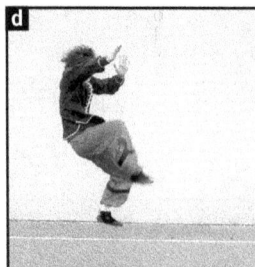

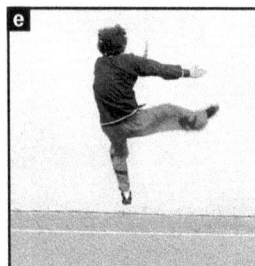

三七、旋風腿

37 - Tornado kick.

Lift up your left leg, and drop the left hand down in a clockwise motion. Then swing up your left leg in a clockwise motion, followed by the kick of the right leg in a clockwise motion. Slap the left side of the right foot with the palm of the left hand.

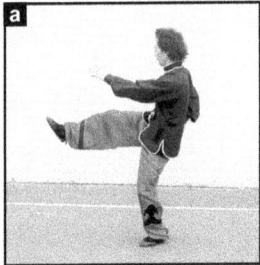

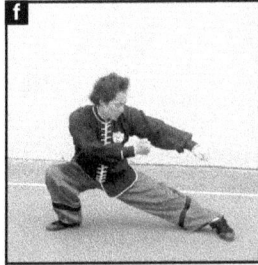

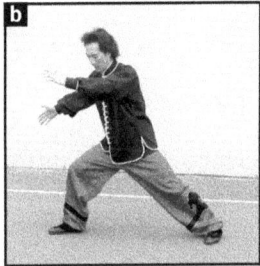

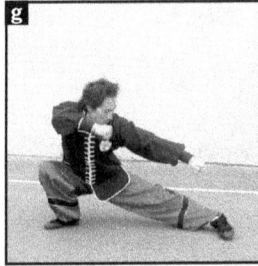

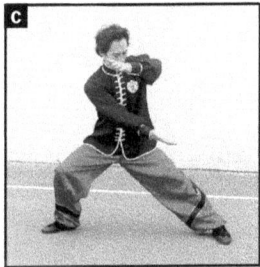

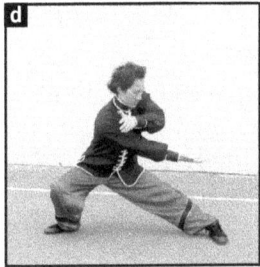

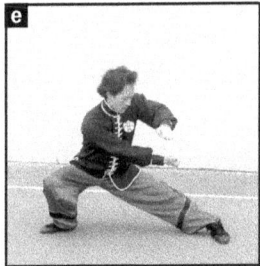

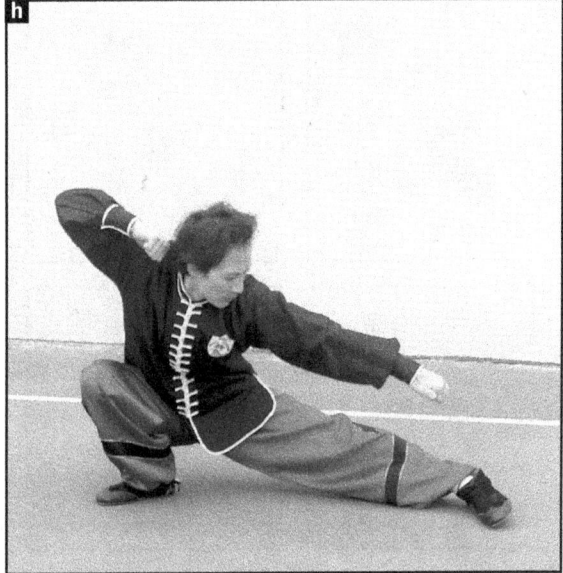

三八、彎弓射虎撲腿勢

38 - Pull the bow. Shoot the tiger. Scattered stance.

First, you will land on your left leg, and then your weight will shift to the right leg. As your weight shifts to the right leg, reach your right hand down (palm up), and bring your left open hand to above your right shoulder.

As you drop the weight onto the left leg and shift in to a left scattered stance, the right hand will pull back and the left hand will punch downward. The left fist will end above the left shin, and the right fist will be to the right side of your head.

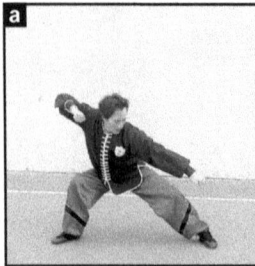

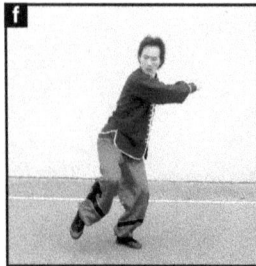

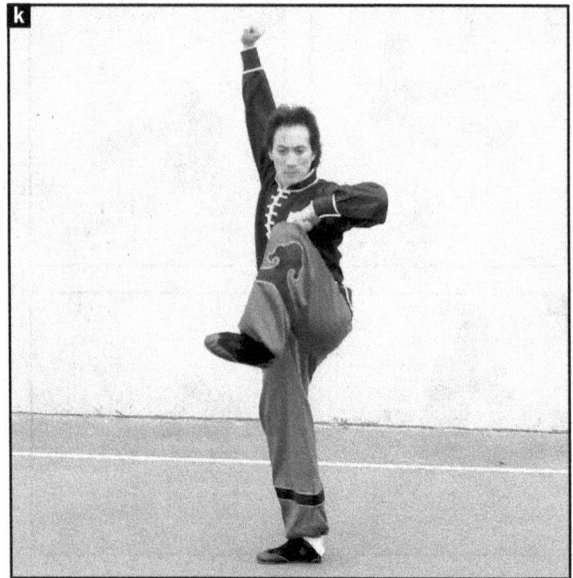

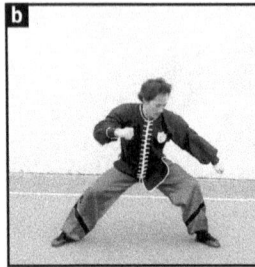

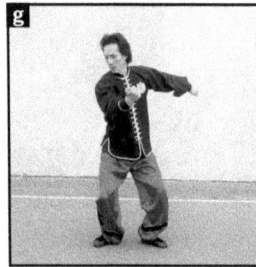

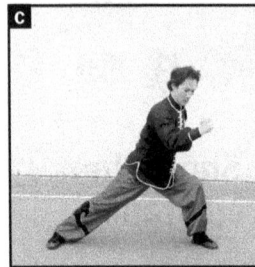

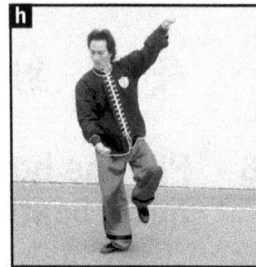

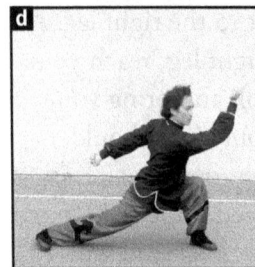

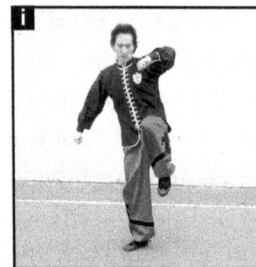

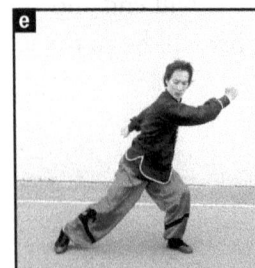

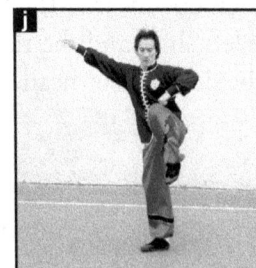

三九、英雄獨立打虎式

39 - Hero stands on one leg. Strike the tiger.

Push off with your right leg and shift into a right bow stance. At the same time, lift the left arm and block down with the outer part of the left forearm, and strike with the inner part of the right forearm using a right to left sideways motion. (**a** to **d**)

Raise your right foot slightly, and as you stamp the ground with the right foot, swing your right hand down, and then up, in a counter-clockwise motion. As the right hand rises up, raise the left leg and the left fist will swing down in a clockwise arc until it rests on top of the left knee.

You may flex the left foot upward (as shown) or you may point your toe downward. Either way is acceptable.

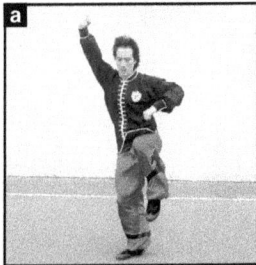

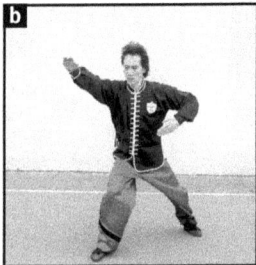

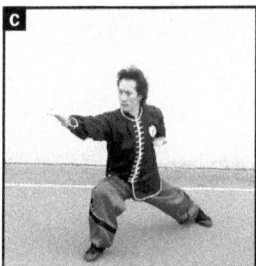

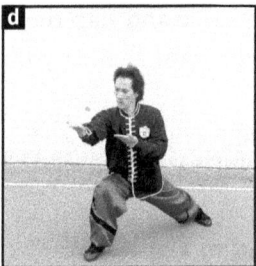

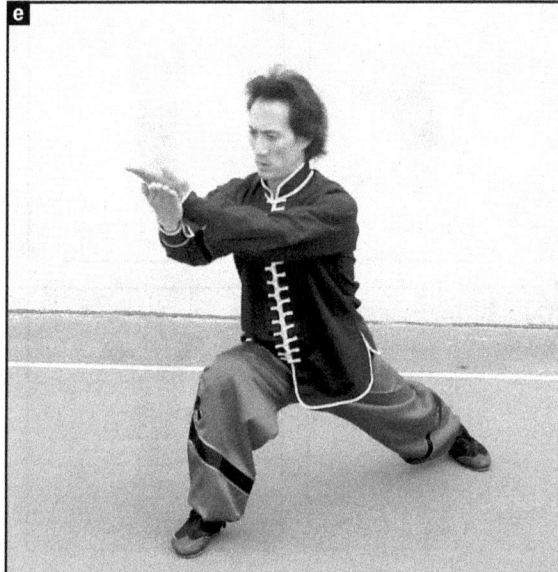

四十、退步穿掌

40A - Step back. Thrust palm.

As the left foot steps back at a 45-degree angle from the right foot, open the right hand (palm up) and drop it down to your right side. Simultaneously, withdraw the left hand to the left side of your body (palm up). You will be in a right bow stance. Thrust the left fingertips forward so that the back of the left hand brushes past the palm of the right hand. This is the piercing palm movement.

Personally, I think of this move as part of the closing bow, but others will think of this move in terms of its application.

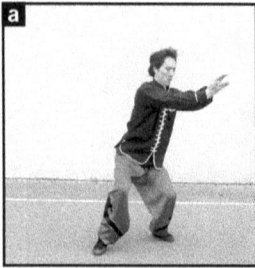

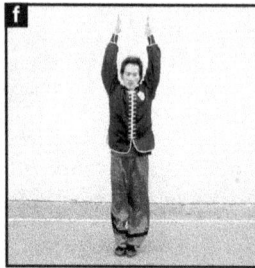

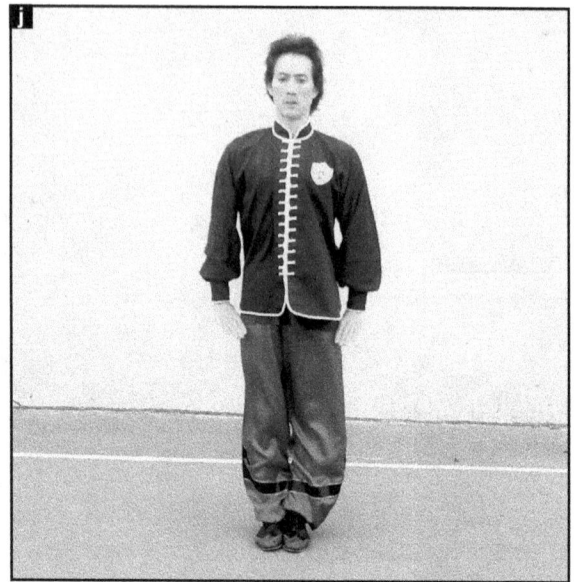

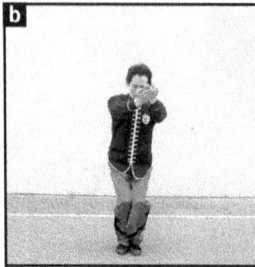

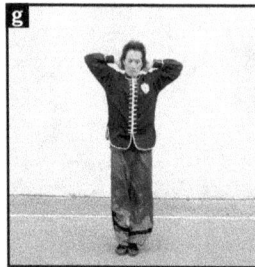

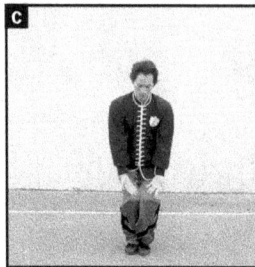

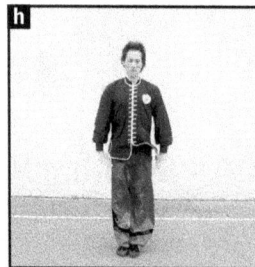

四十、 收 式

40B - Finishing posture.

Then, step back with the right foot and bring the right foot alongside the left foot. Bring both hands to the middle and slap the outsides of your palms downward against your thighs. (**a** to **c**)

Bring the arms all the way up.

Push down with both palms. Bow, and then raise the upper torso so you are upright. The set is now complete. (**d** to **f**)

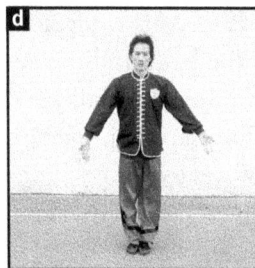

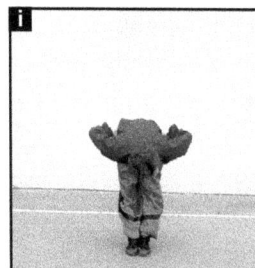

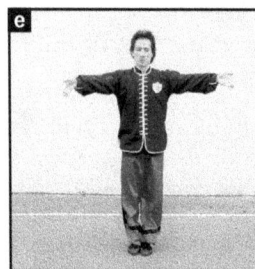

74

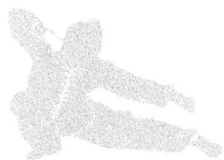

Shaolin #8: Uprooting Step - Back Views

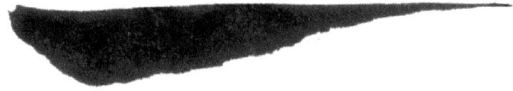

Shaolin #8: Uprooting Step - Back Views

The following set of photos show the movements as back views. This is how they would appear to someone standing behind an instructor. The numbers match the front view photos given in the earlier section of the book.

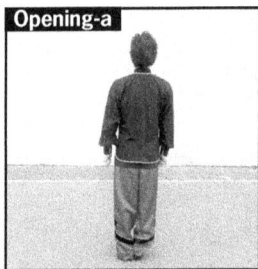

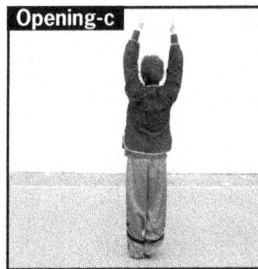

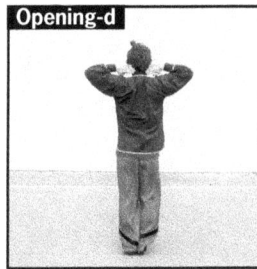

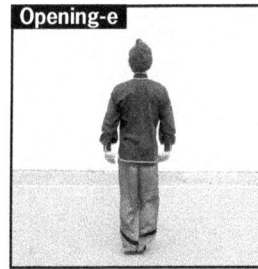

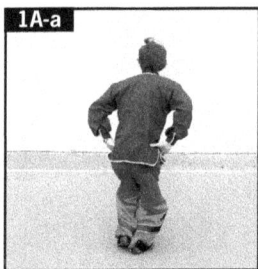

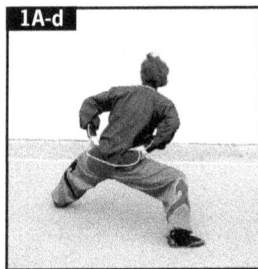

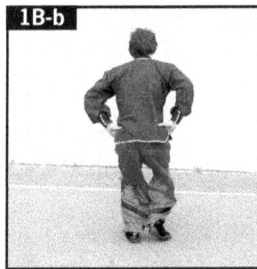

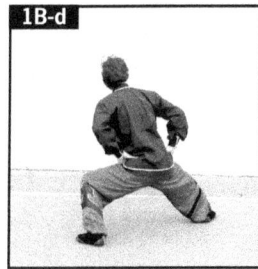

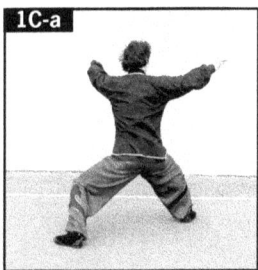

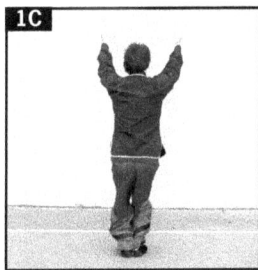

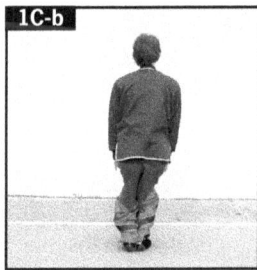

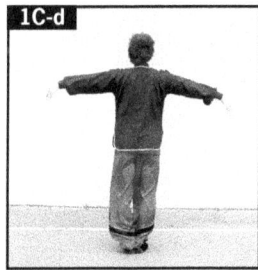

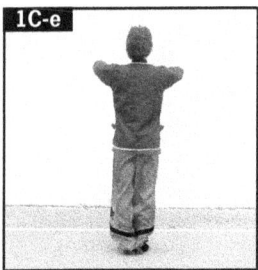

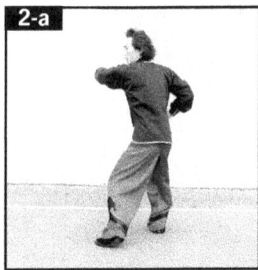

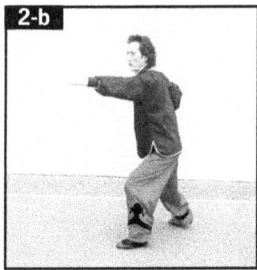

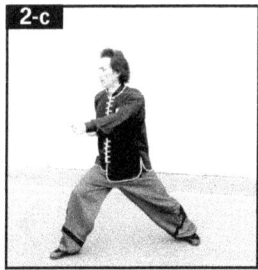

Opening-a | Opening-c | Opening-d | Opening-e

1A-a | 1A-d | 1B-b | 1B-d

1C-a | 1C | 1C-b | 1C-d

1C-e | 2-a | 2-b | 2-c

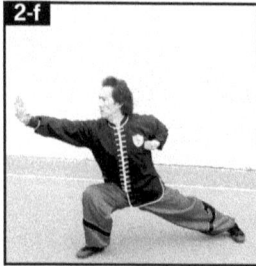
2-f

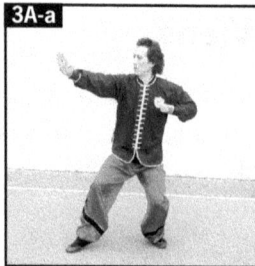
3A-a

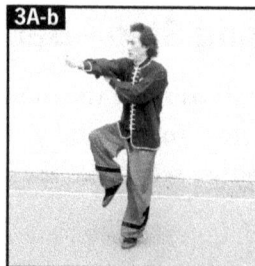
3A-b

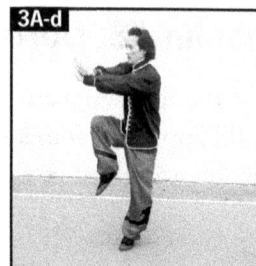
3A-d

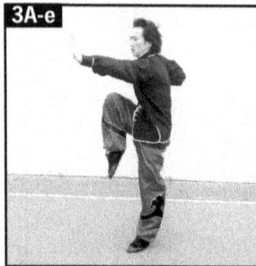
3A-e

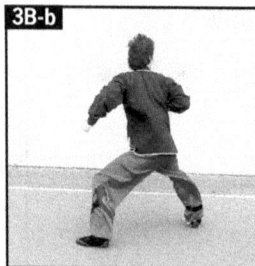
3B-b

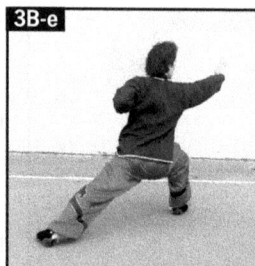
3B-e

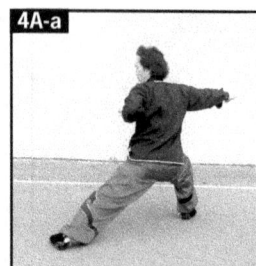
4A-a

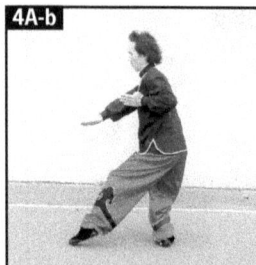
4A-b

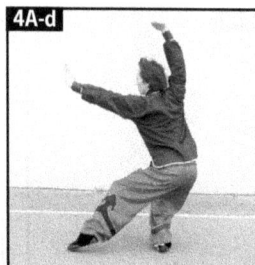
4A-d

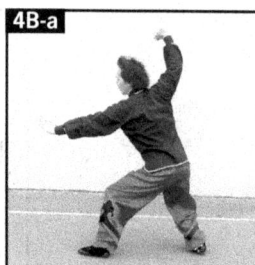
4B-a

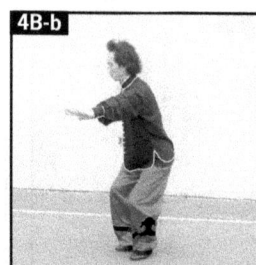
4B-b

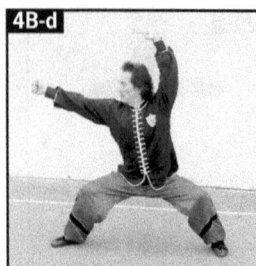
4B-d

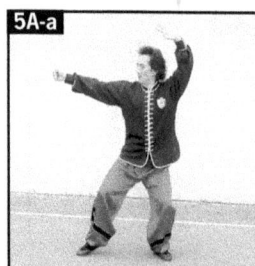
5A-a

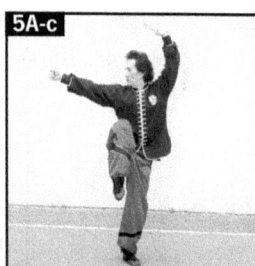
5A-c

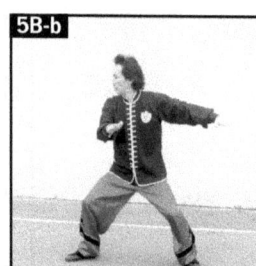
5B-b

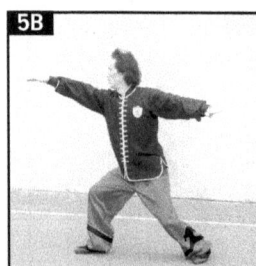
5B

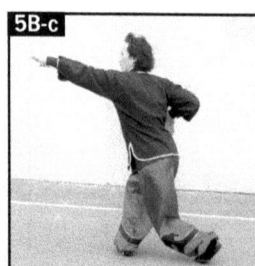
5B-c

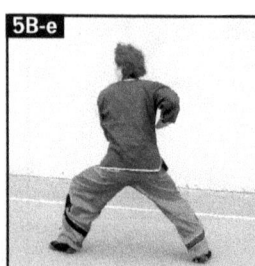
5B-e

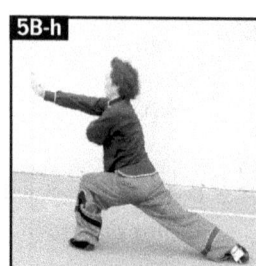
5B-h

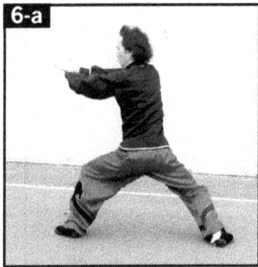

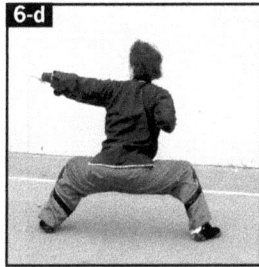

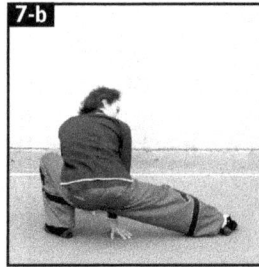

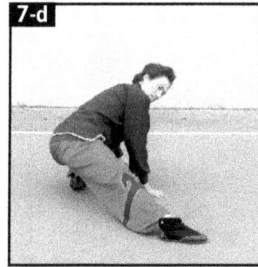

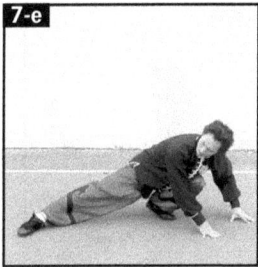

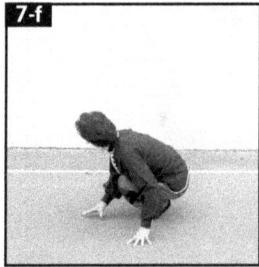

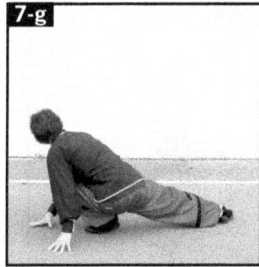

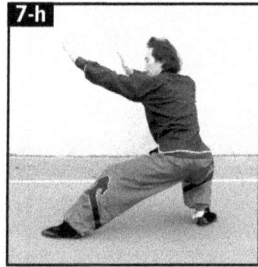

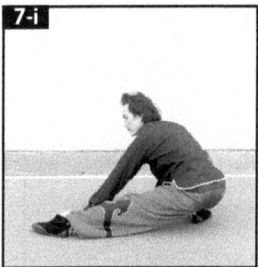

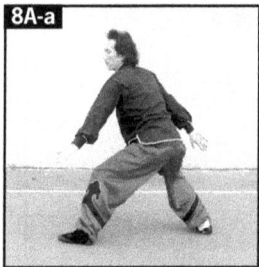

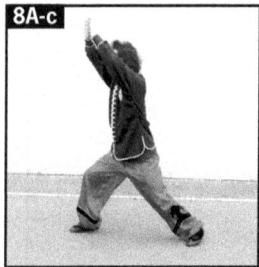

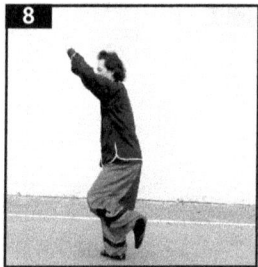

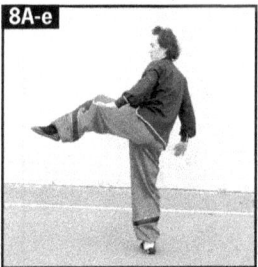

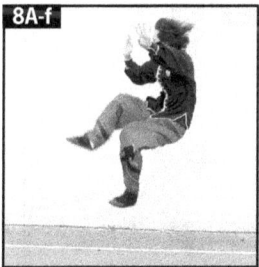

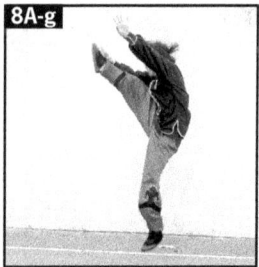

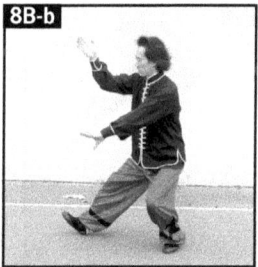

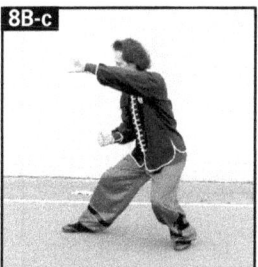

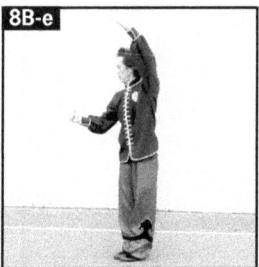

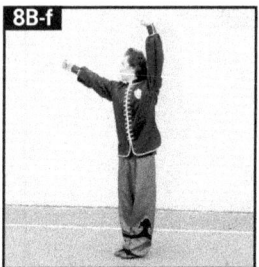

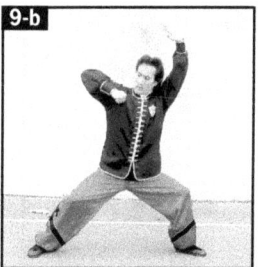

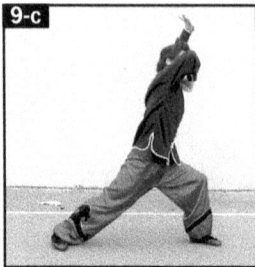
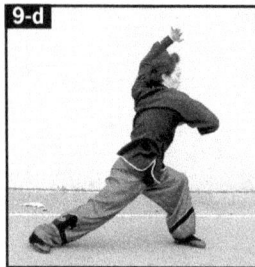
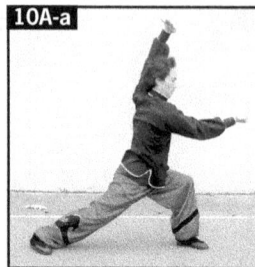
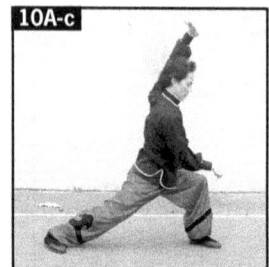
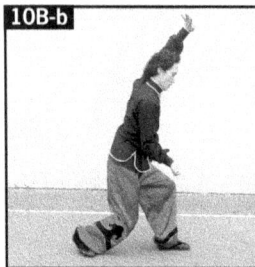
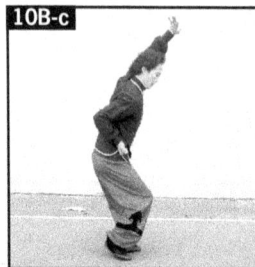
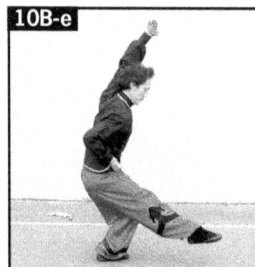
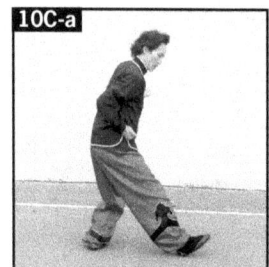
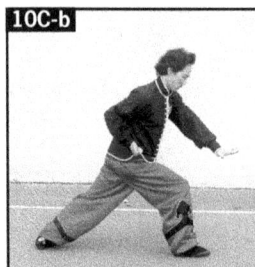
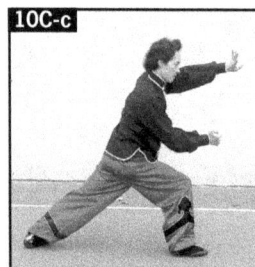
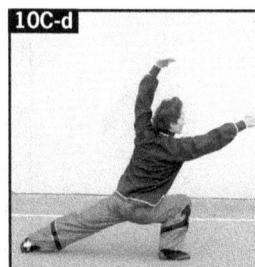
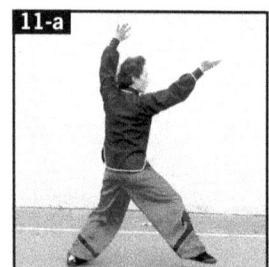
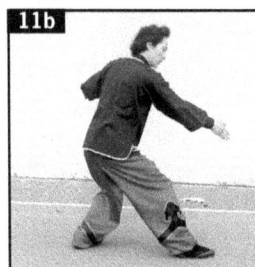
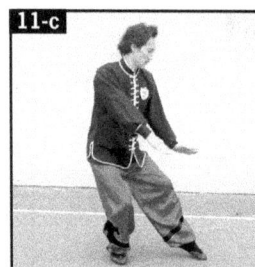
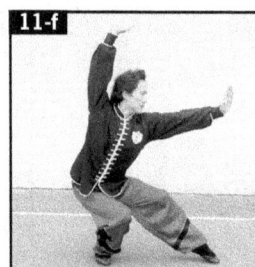
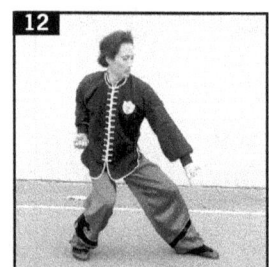
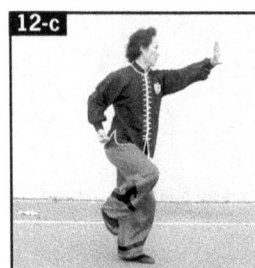
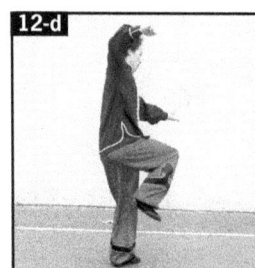
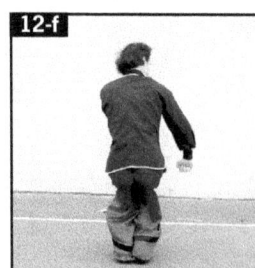
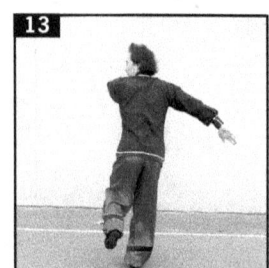

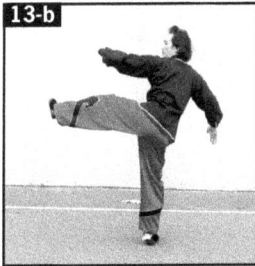
13-b

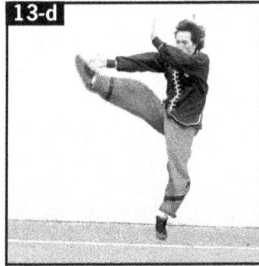
13-d

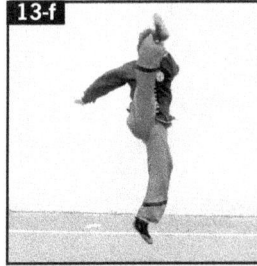
13-f

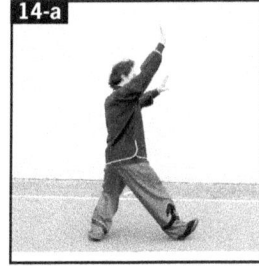
14-a

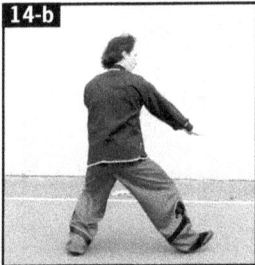
14-b

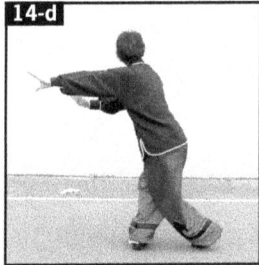
14-d

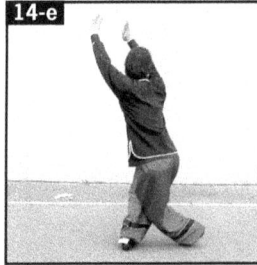
14-e

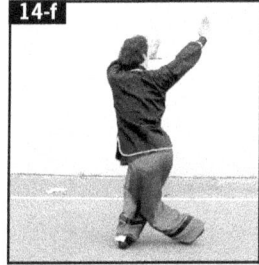
14-f

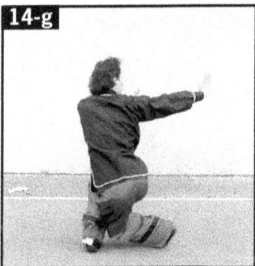
14-g

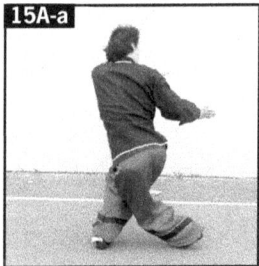
15A-a

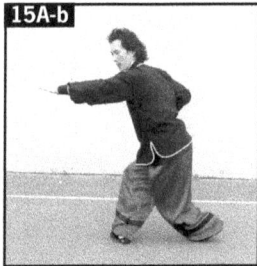
15A-b

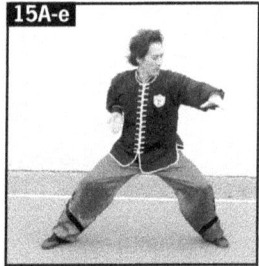
15A-e

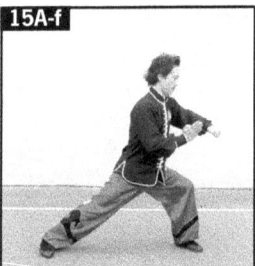
15A-f

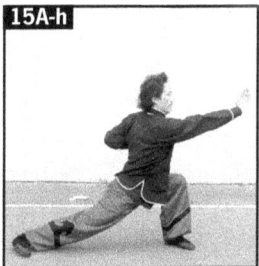
15A-h

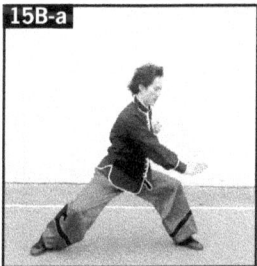
15B-a

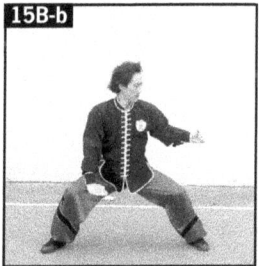
15B-b

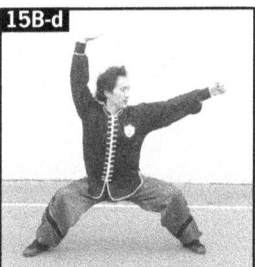
15B-d

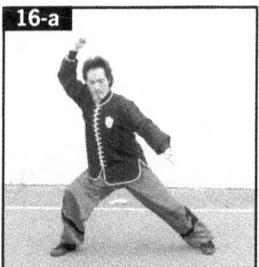
16-a

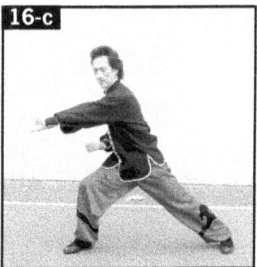
16-c

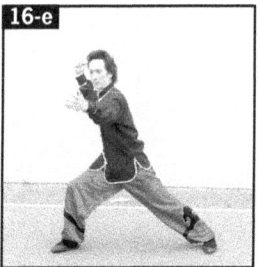
16-e

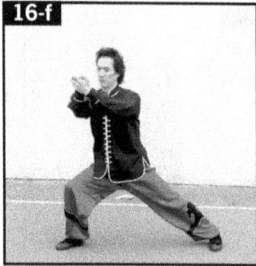
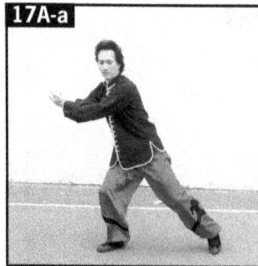
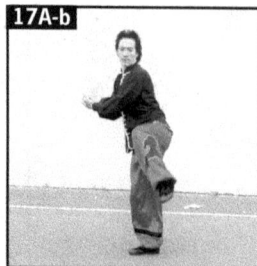
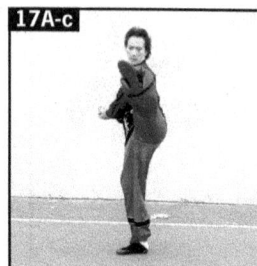
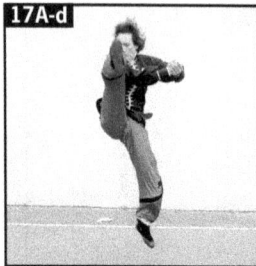
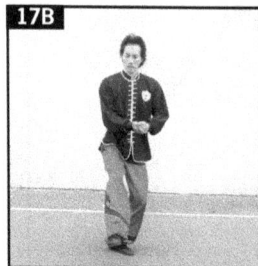
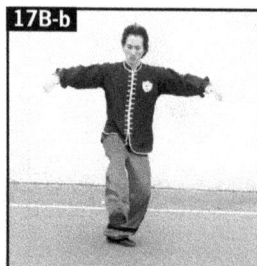
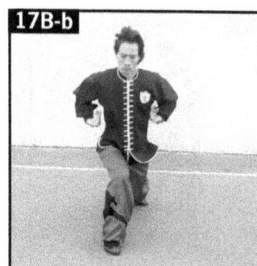
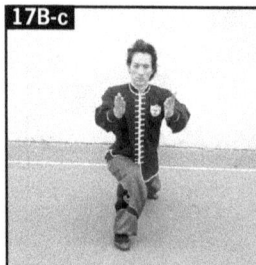
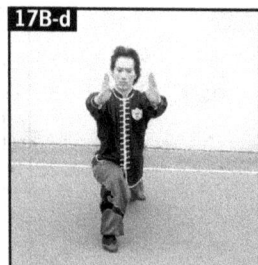
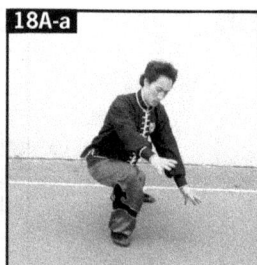
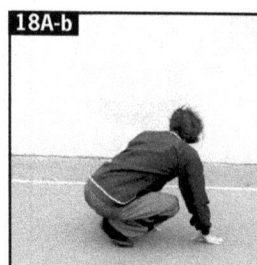
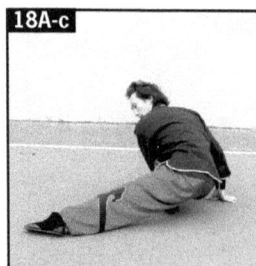
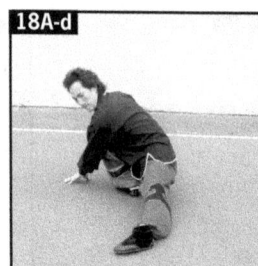
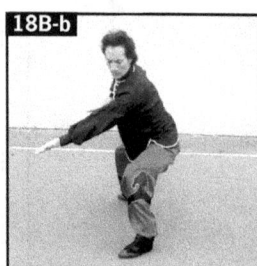
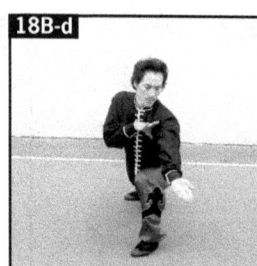
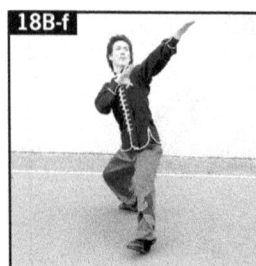
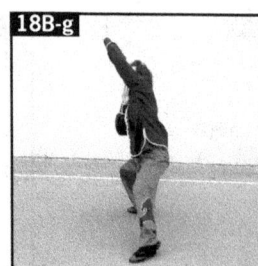
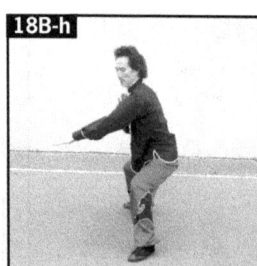
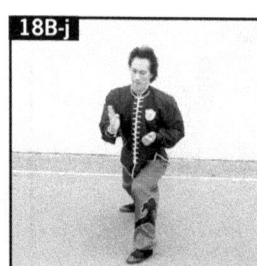

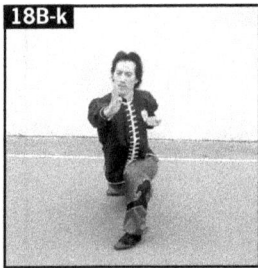
18B-k

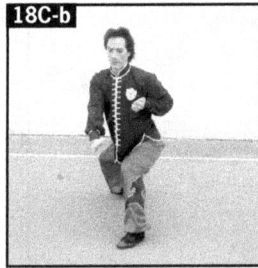
18C-b

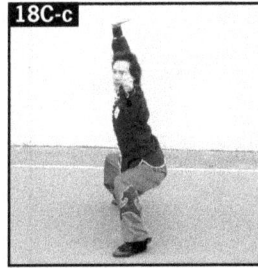
18C-c

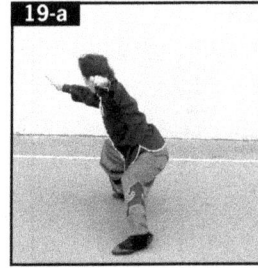
19-a

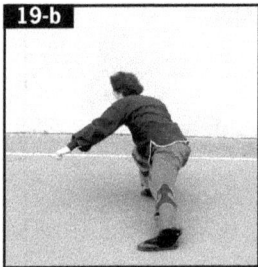
19-b

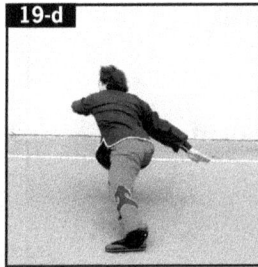
19-d

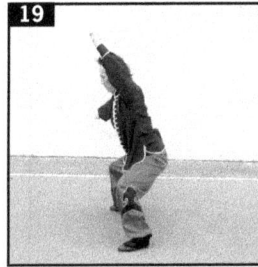
19

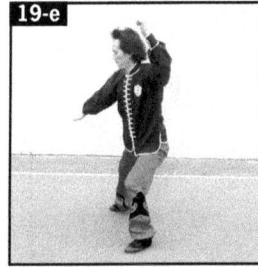
19-e

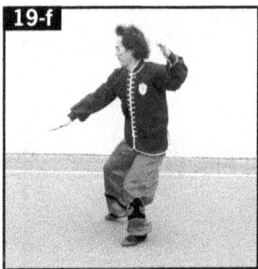
19-f

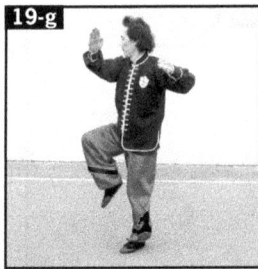
19-g

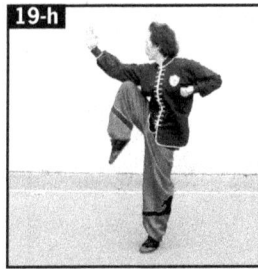
19-h

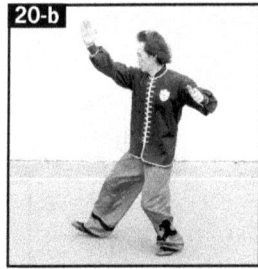
20-b

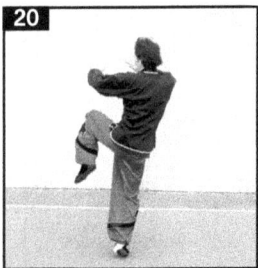
20

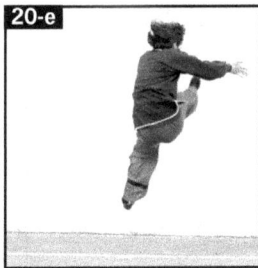
20-e

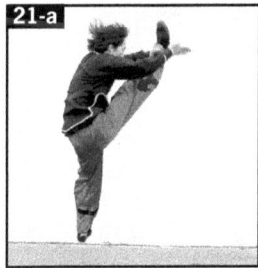
21-a

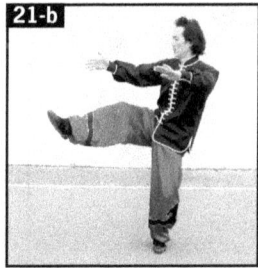
21-b

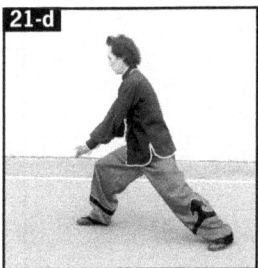
21-d

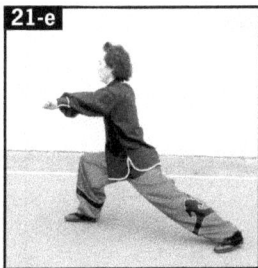
21-e

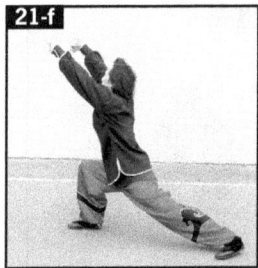
21-f

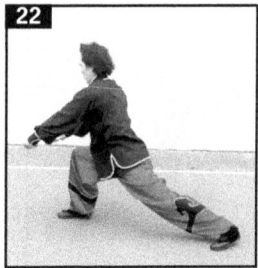
22

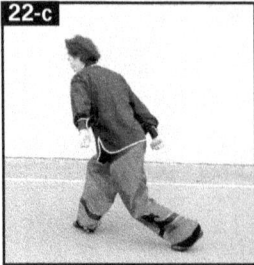

22-c

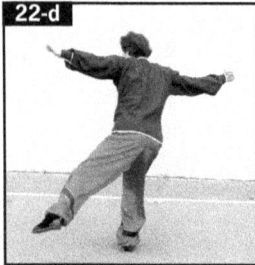

22-d

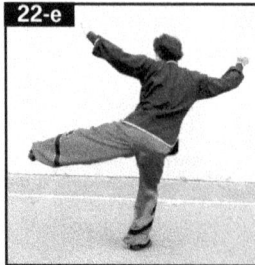

22-e

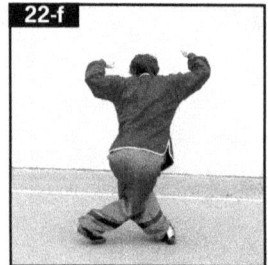

22-f

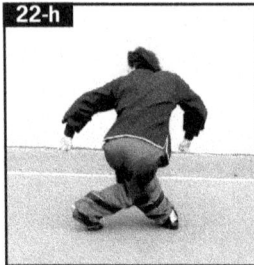

22-h

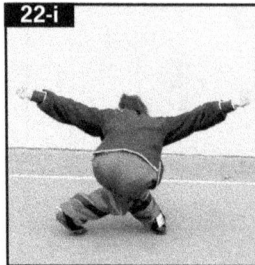

22-i

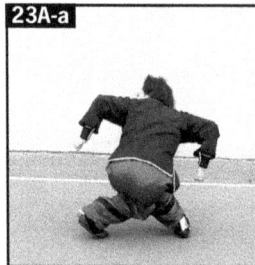

23A-a

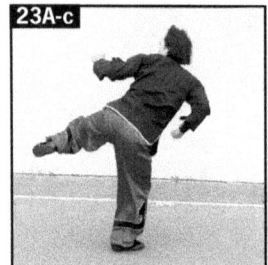

23A-c

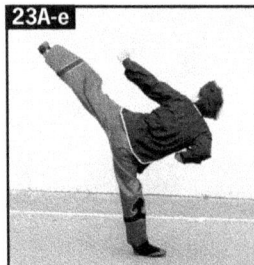

23A-e

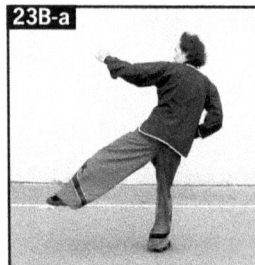

23B-a

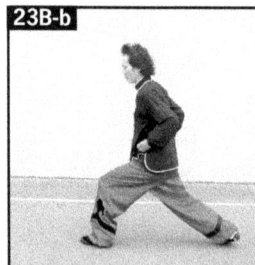

23B-b

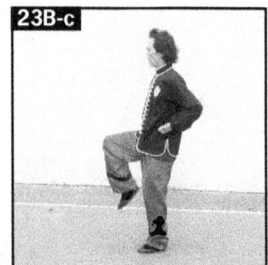

23B-c

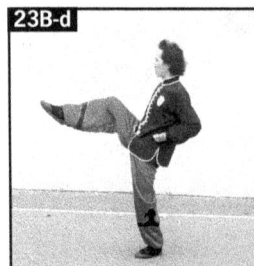

23B-d

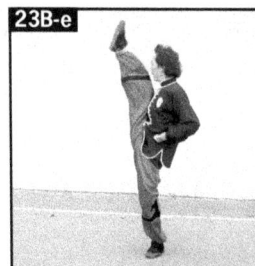

23B-e

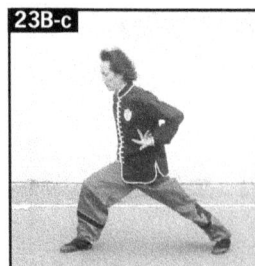

23B-c

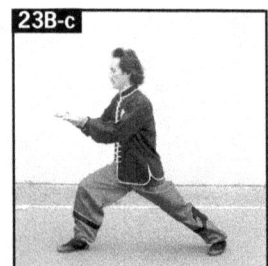

23B-c

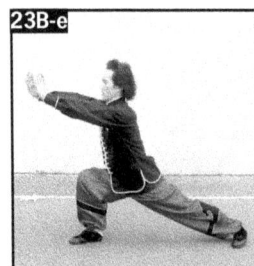

23B-e

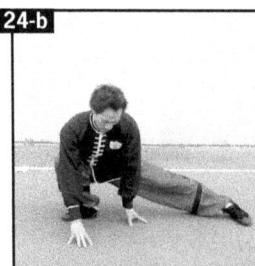

24-b

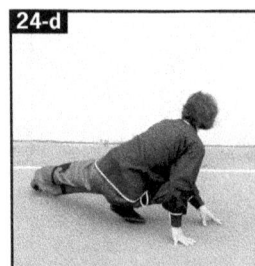

24-d

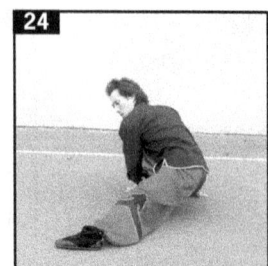

24

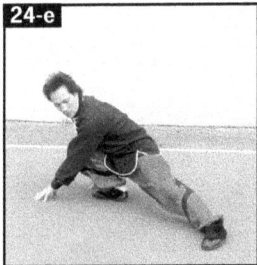

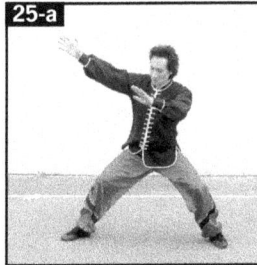

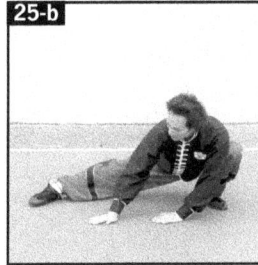

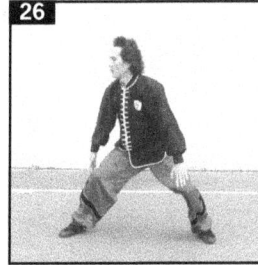

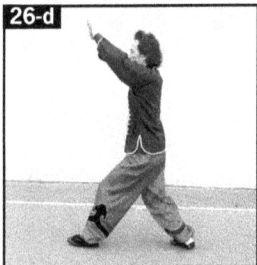

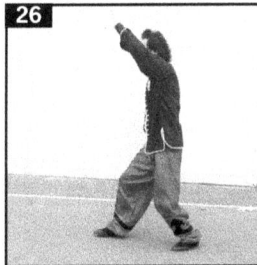

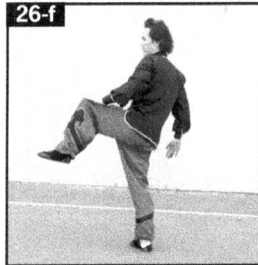

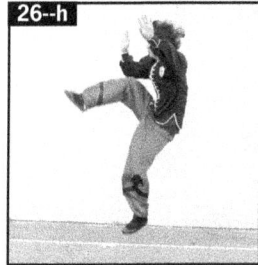

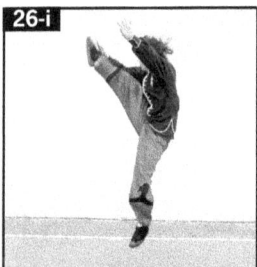

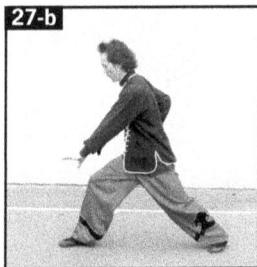

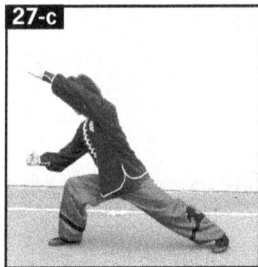

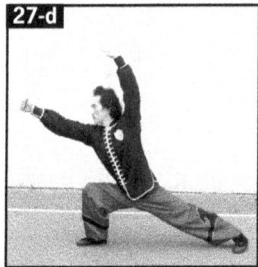

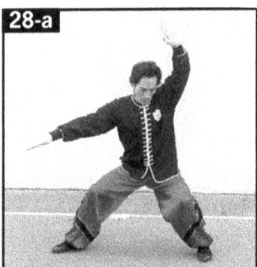

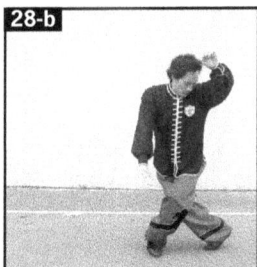

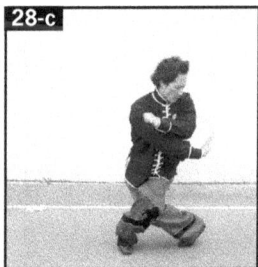

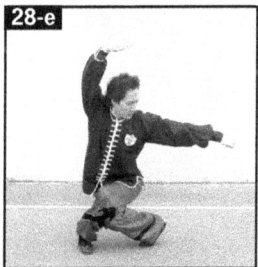

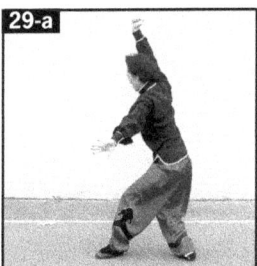

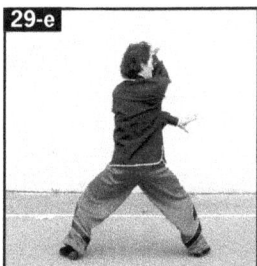

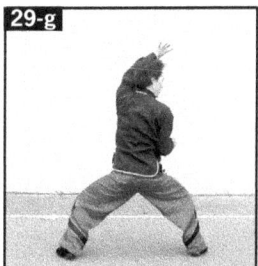

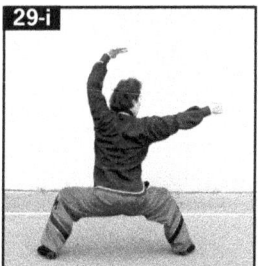

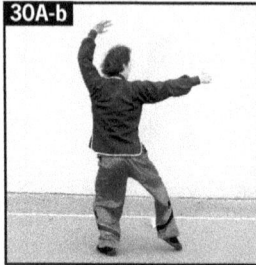
30A-b

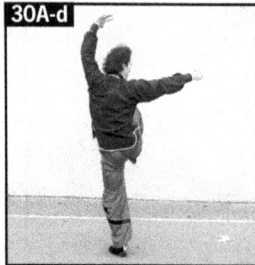
30A-d

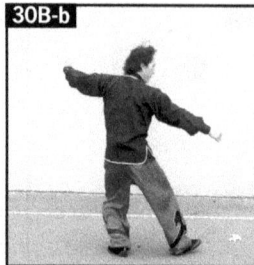
30B-b

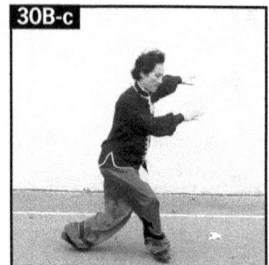
30B-c

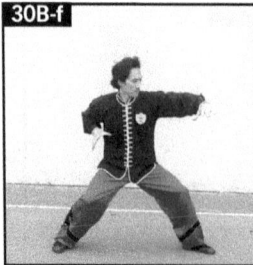
30B-f

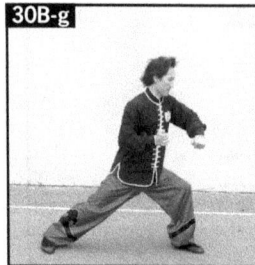
30B-g

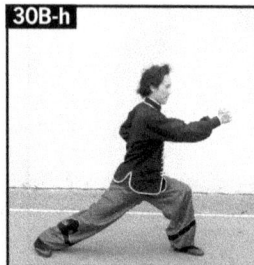
30B-h

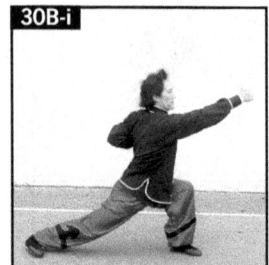
30B-i

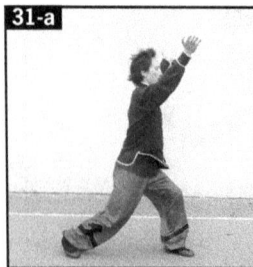
31-a

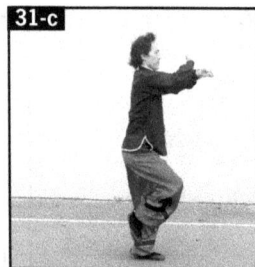
31-c

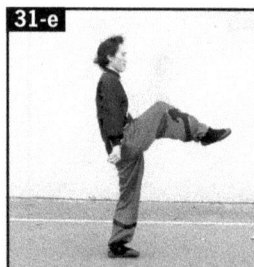
31-e

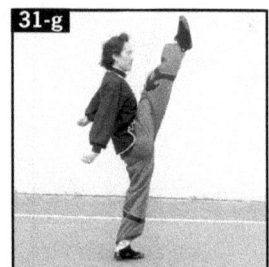
31-g

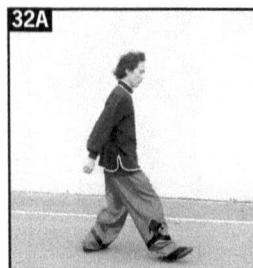
32A

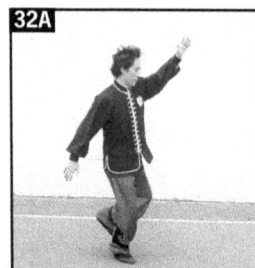
32A

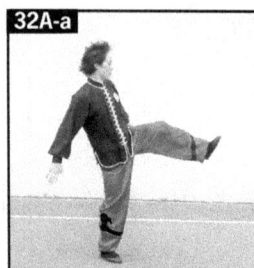
32A-a

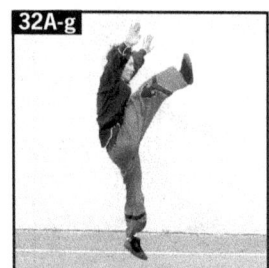
32A-g

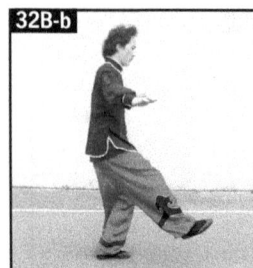
32B-b

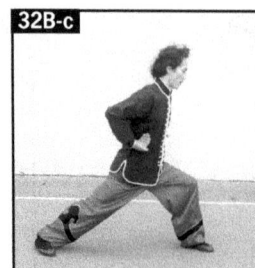
32B-c

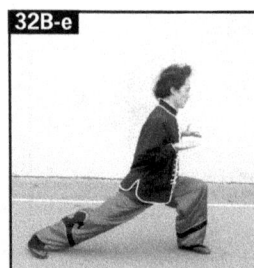
32B-e

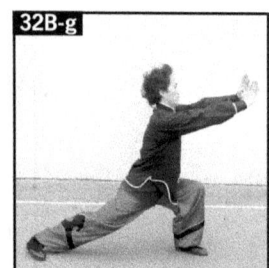
32B-g

88

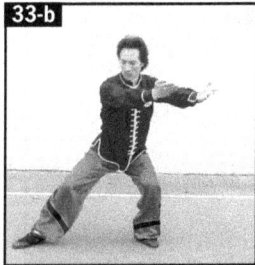
33-b

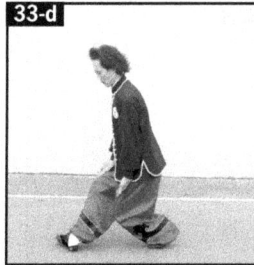
33-d

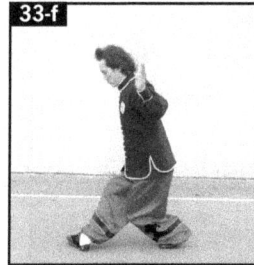
33-f

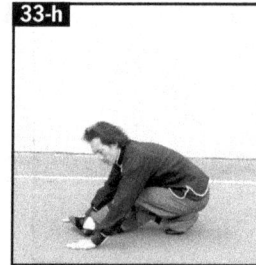
33-h

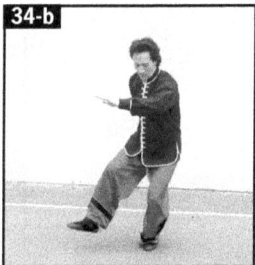
34-b

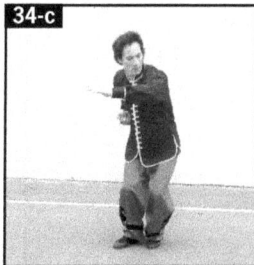
34-c

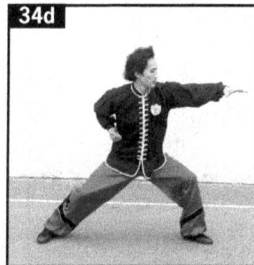
34d

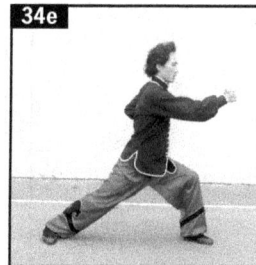
34e

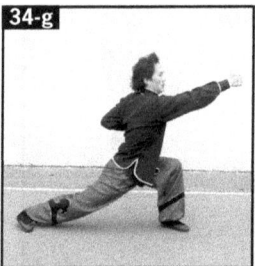
34-g

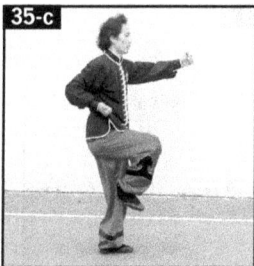
35-c

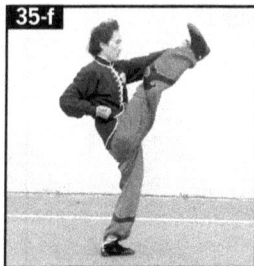
35-f

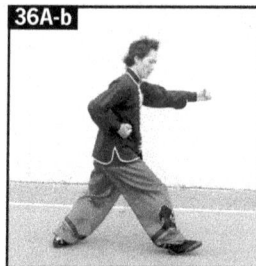
36A-b

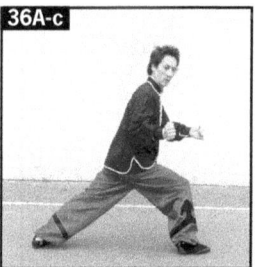
36A-c

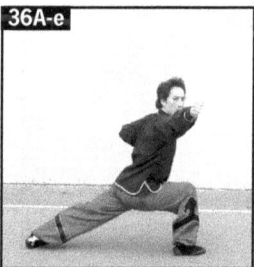
36A-e

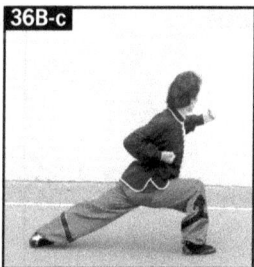
36B-c

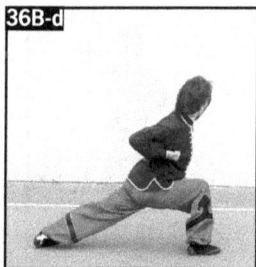
36B-d

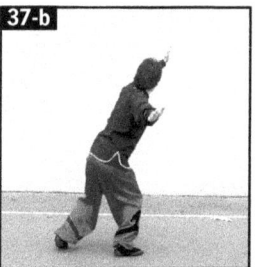
37-b

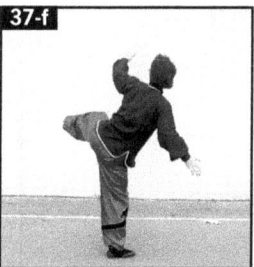
37-f

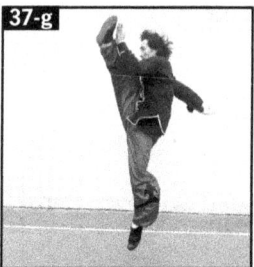
37-g

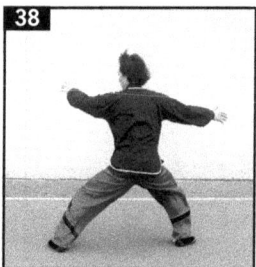
38

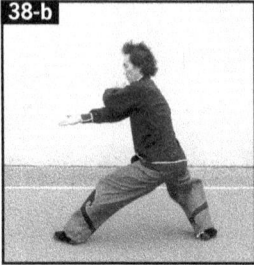
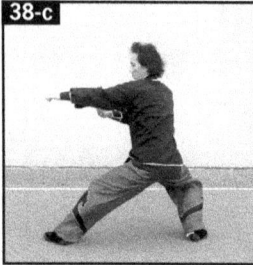
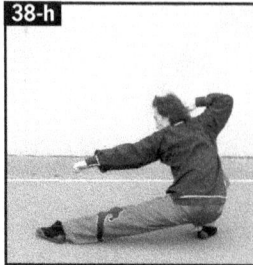
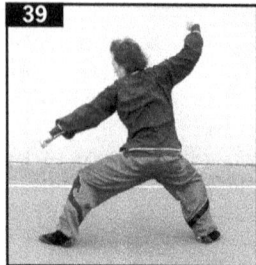
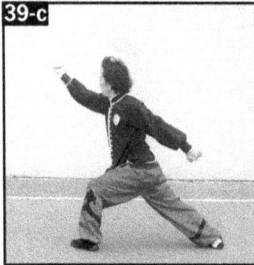
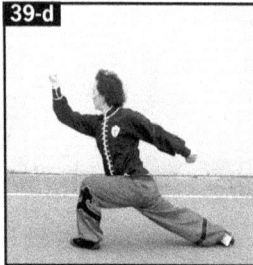
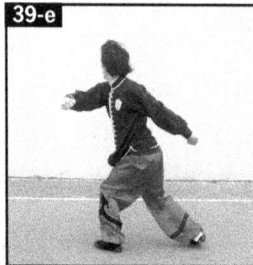
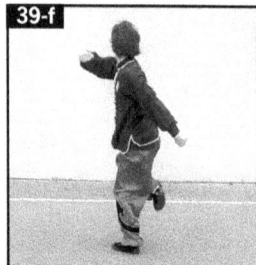
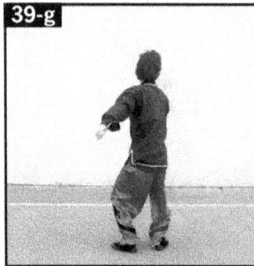
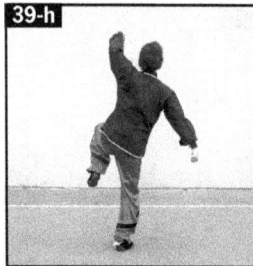
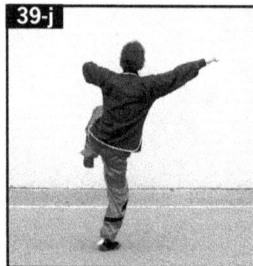
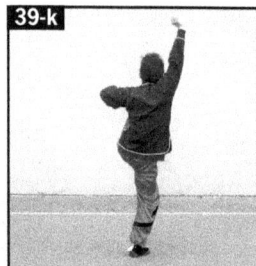
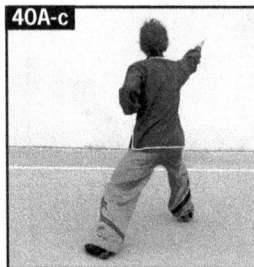
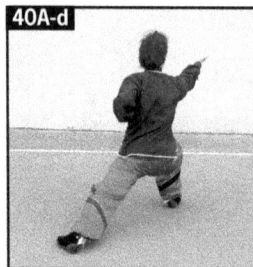
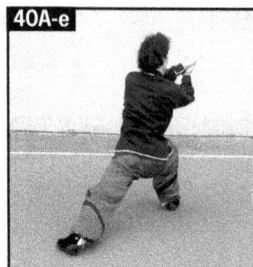
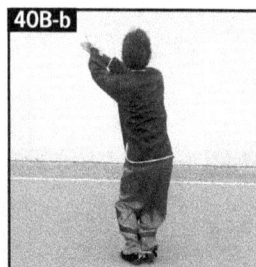
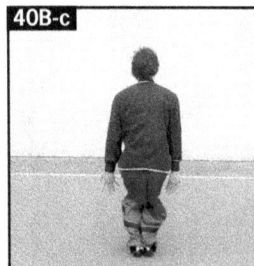
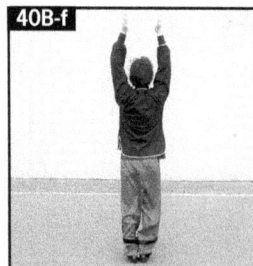
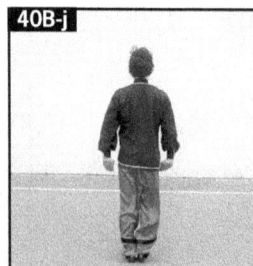

Shaolin #8: Selected Applications

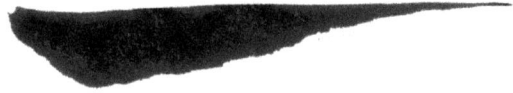

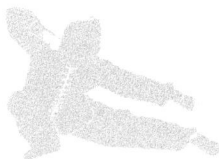

Shaolin #8: Selected Applications

This section shows basic applications of the movements in Shaolin #8, and closely follows the movements of the set itself. For most of the movements, I will show only one application, although many are possible.

Be careful not to get overly fancy with the applications. Simpler is better, and my teacher, Sifu Wong Jack Man, always emphasized simplicity over complexity.

1A - Immortal shakes his clothes. Step forward.

Use the left leg to break the opponent's horse stance by sweeping forward. These photos show the breaking of his horse stance from the inside. You may also use your left hand to tug at him so as to steady yourself and make your sweep seem even more powerful. You may also use your left hand to grab his arm or shoulder and pull him off balance.

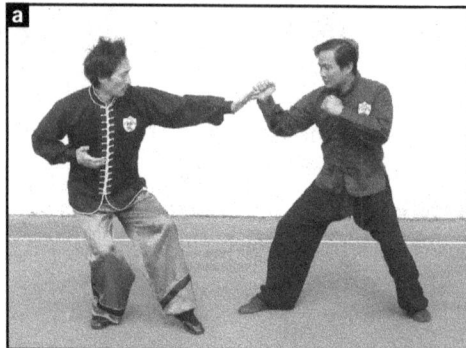

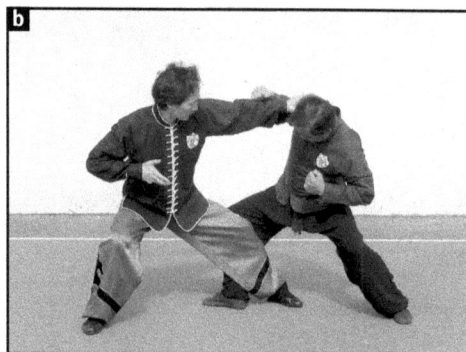

1A alternate

As an alternative, you may use the left leg to break the opponent's horse from the outside.

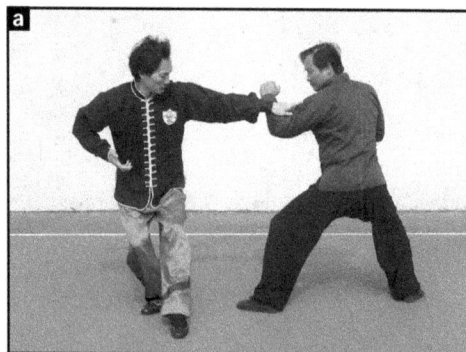

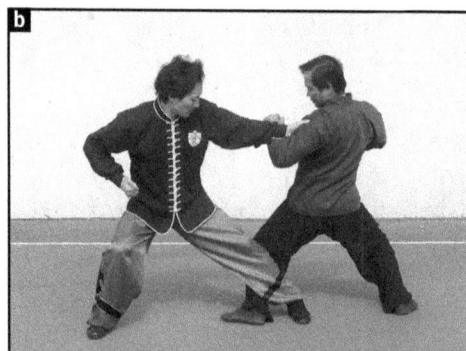

1B -   Step forward.

Similarly, you may use the right leg to break the opponent's horse from the inside.

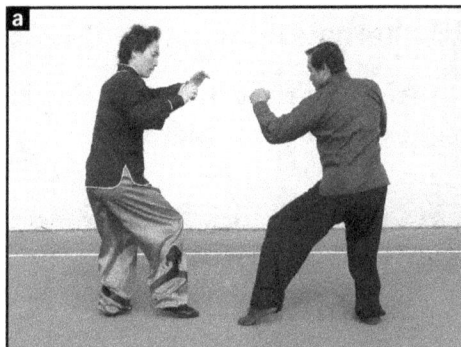

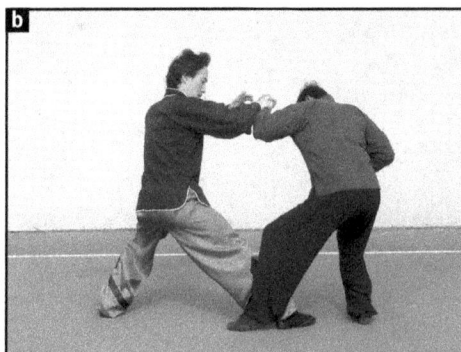

1B alternate

Use your right leg to step in and break his horse from the outside.

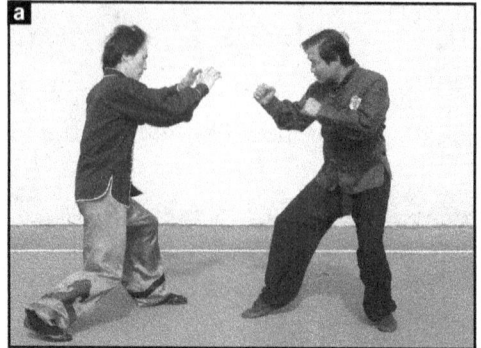

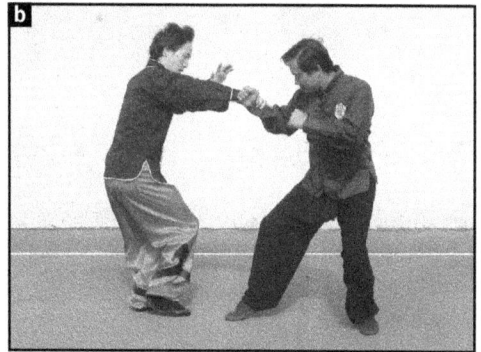

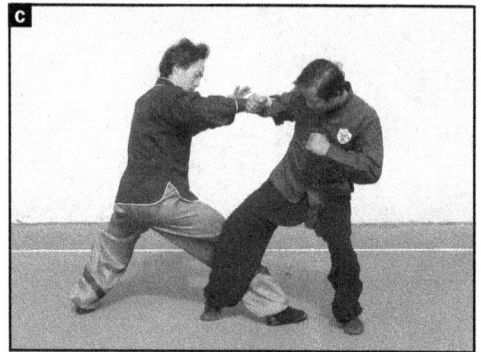

1C - Double matching fists.

If the opponent puts both of his hands on my shoulders to grab me, I can brush downward with the back of my hands to remove his hands. Then, I continue the circular motion of my hands and strike him in the chest. Many times, movements are done in the set with both hands for symmetry and exercise purposes, but the applications can be done with both hands, or, simply with one hand, depending on the situation.

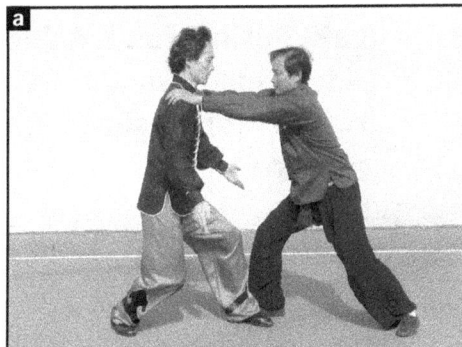

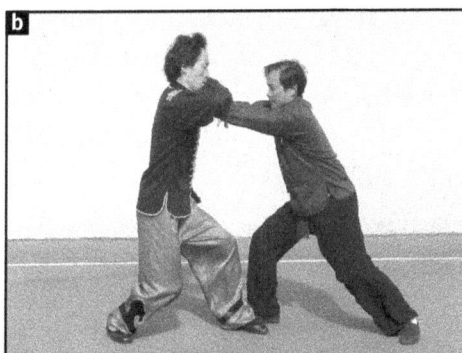

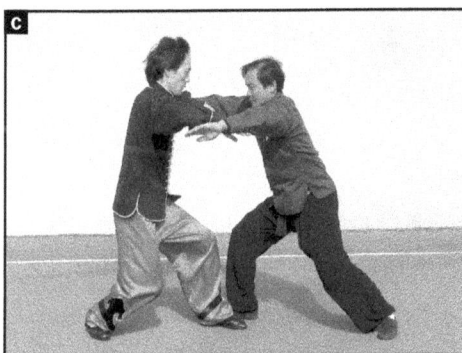

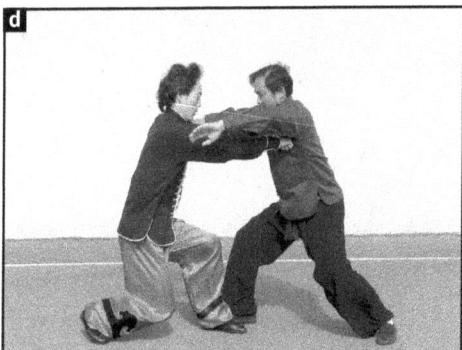

2 - (Left) Pulling Hand. Angled (side) step. Advance with a (right) cutting palm in a right bow stance.

If the opponent attempts to strike me with his left hand, I grab it with my left hand and strike him in the head with my right palm. Strike whatever opening is available to you. If the opponent is very tall, you may strike him in the chest instead. Notice that this is a very basic motion, and because the motion is so basic, there are a myriad of applications.

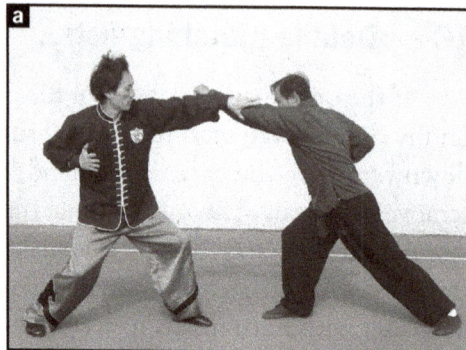

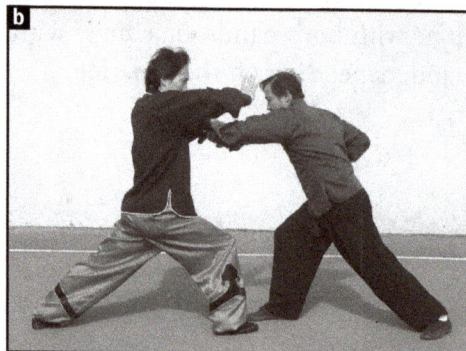

3A - Step back. (Right leg up, left palm).

Pull his hand inward in with your right hand, and strike him with your left palm. Use a knee strike at the same time so that you may maximize your chance of hitting him.

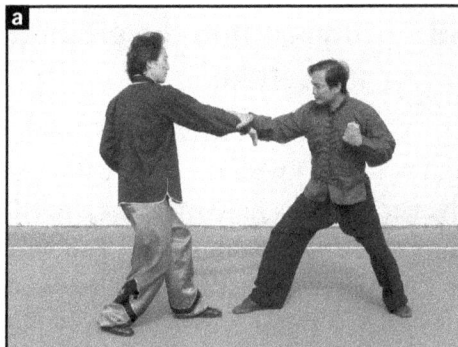

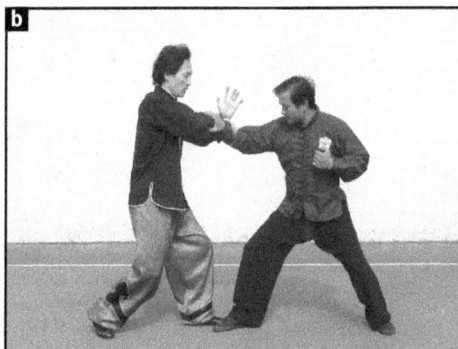

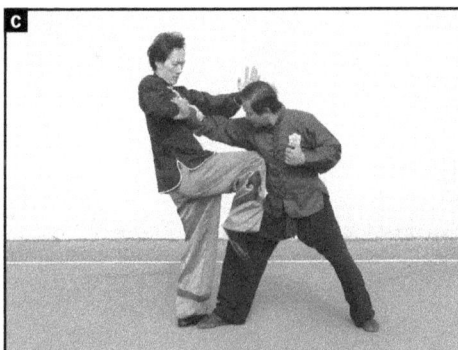

3B - "Uppercut to the groin" (right) palm strike.

Clear away his strike with your left hand, and strike him with the right palm. Although the name of this movement is "Uppercut to the groin (right) palm strike," I show a strike to the opponent's head. Of course, you may also strike lower if the opportunity presents itself.

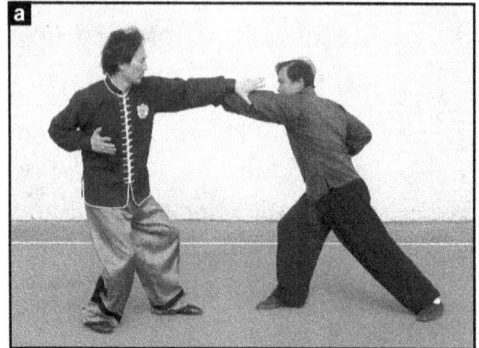

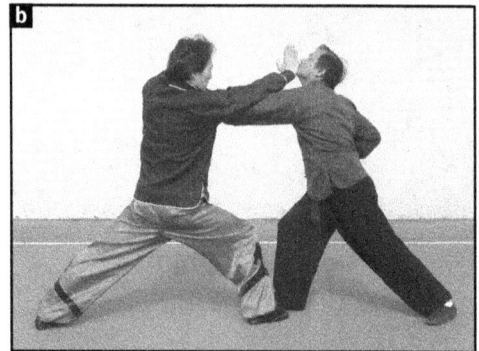

4A - Step forward (Left cat stance).
Lift hands. (Left palm strike).

I parry his strike upward with my right hand, and strike him under the chin with the fingertips of my left hand.

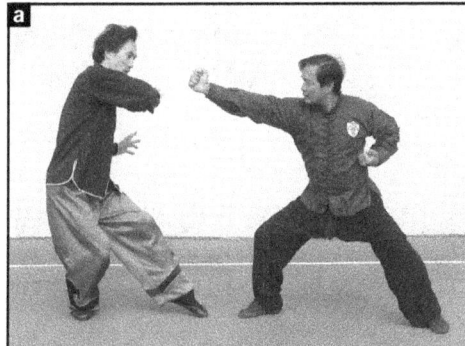

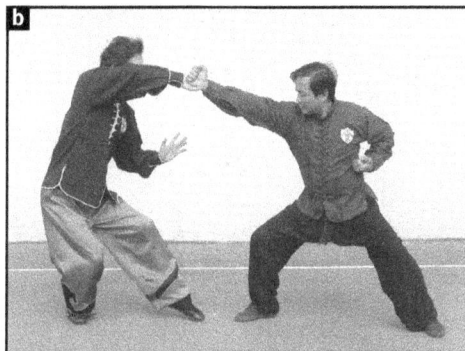

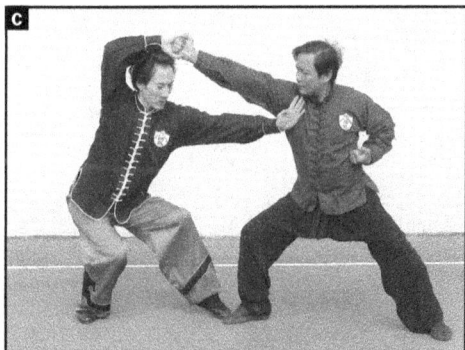

4A alternate

Alternatively, I could block his strike upward and attack his groin.

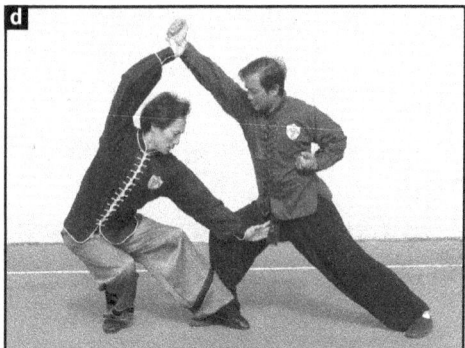

4B - Sit in horse stance. Block and strike. (Right fist strike).

This is another very basic motion. I guide his strike upward and away with my left hand, and then step in to strike with my right fist.

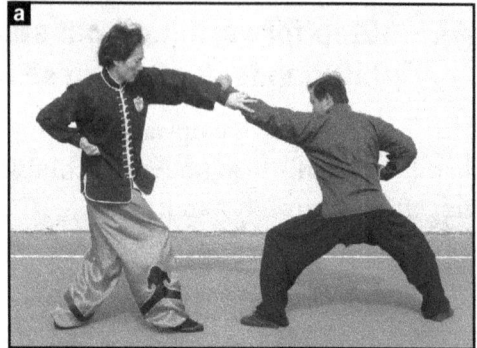

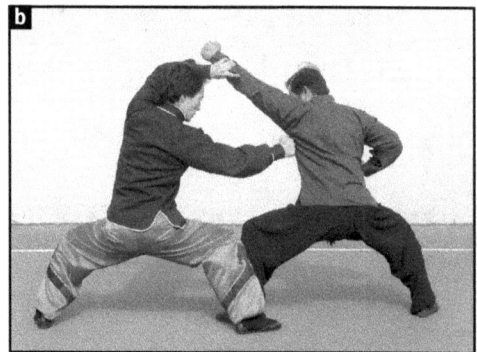

5A - Raise the right leg.

If he attempts to sweep me, I can simply raise my right leg to avoid the sweep. Actually, it really doesn't matter too much which position your hands are in, but I assume a stance similar to that of the form for clarity of the "visual" explanation of this move.

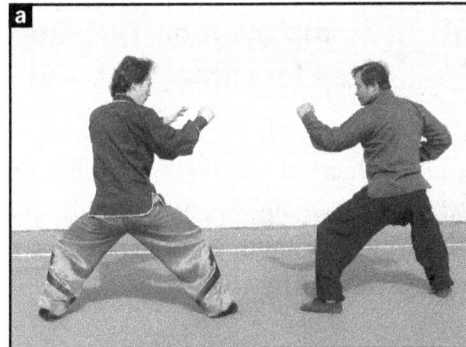

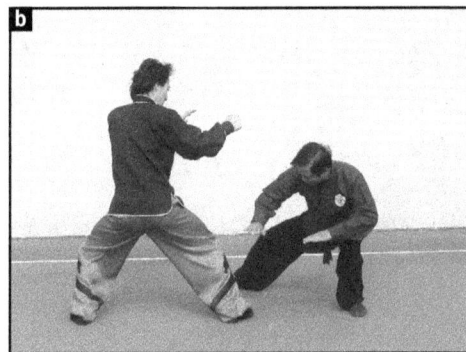

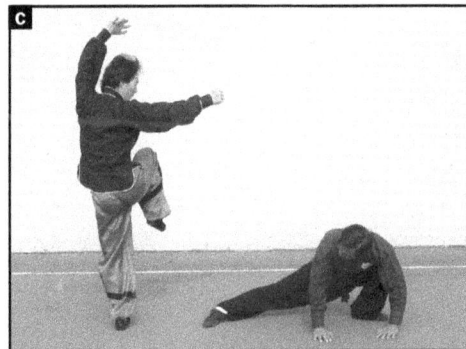

5B - Stamp the foot. Tangling hand. Step forward. Press and strike.

This is another very common move in Chinese martial arts. First, grab his striking arm with your right hand, second, control it with your left hand, and then finally, strike him with your right hand.

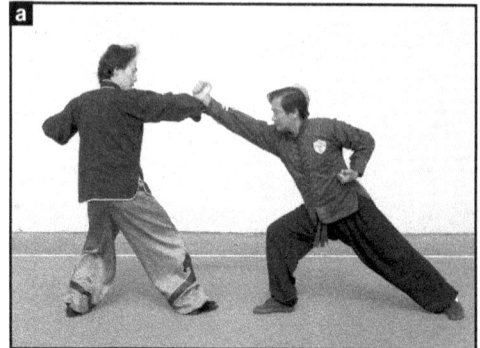

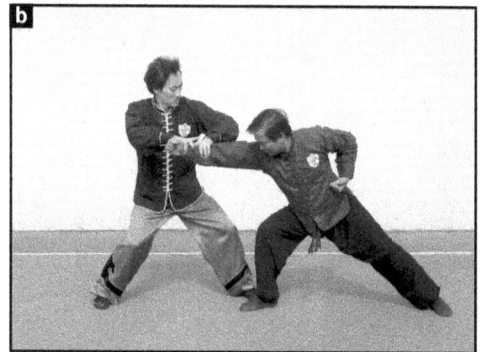

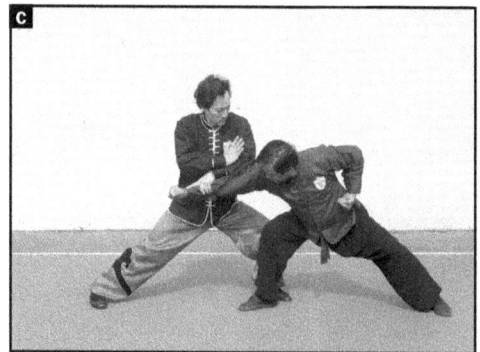

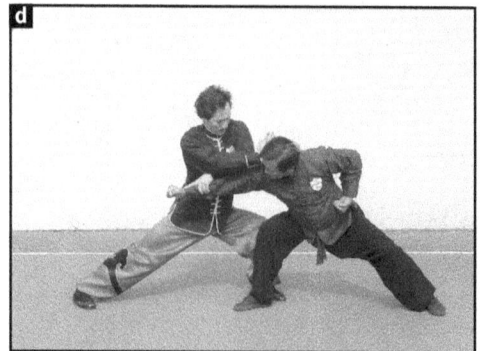

6 - Wipe off the hand. Strike with the palm. Horse stance.

If he attempts to grab your right hand, pull the right arm back and use that pulling force to accentuate the forward slide of your left hand to strike him with even more force.

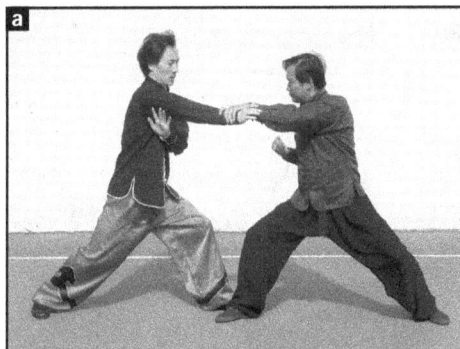

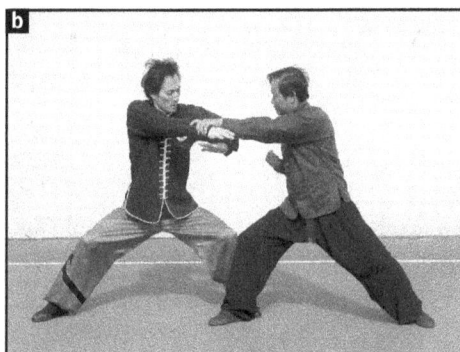

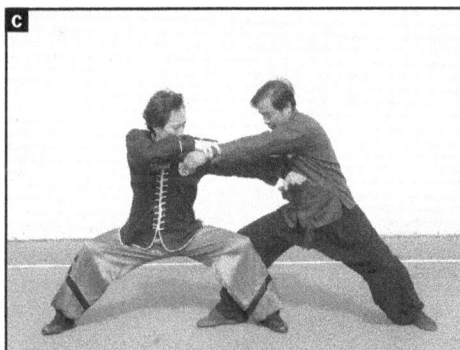

7A - Back sweep.

I show this sweep as a counterattack to a fist strike, although it could also be used against kicks. As he attempts to strike me with his right fist, I use a back sweep with my right leg to knock his right leg out from under him.

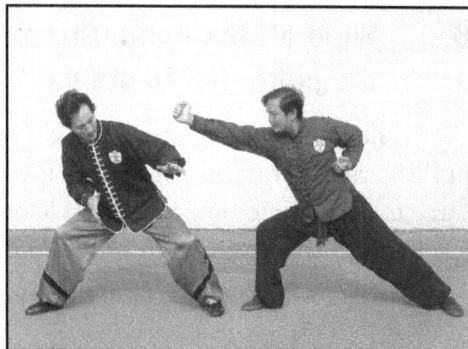

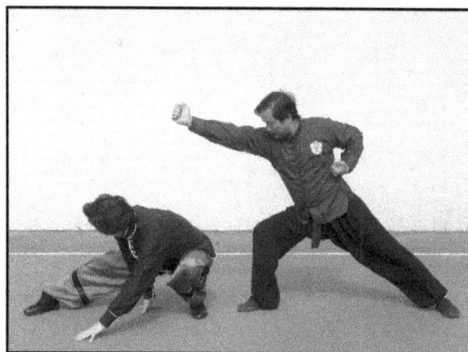

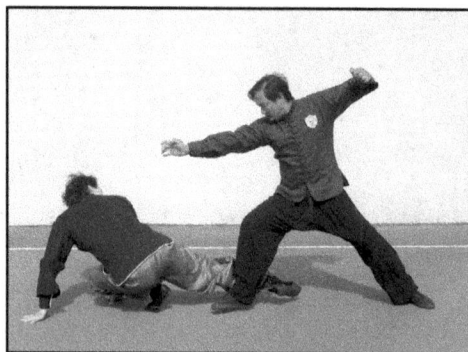

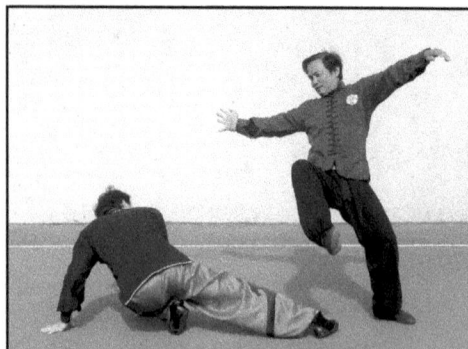

7B - Slap the ground. Flying sand.

As the sweep is being completed, the practitioner is to slap the ground with both hands. This may be used as a precautionary move, and so, if the opponent attempts to kick you after your sweep has missed its target, slap his kick down hard. In this case, slap his kick down to protect your face and body.

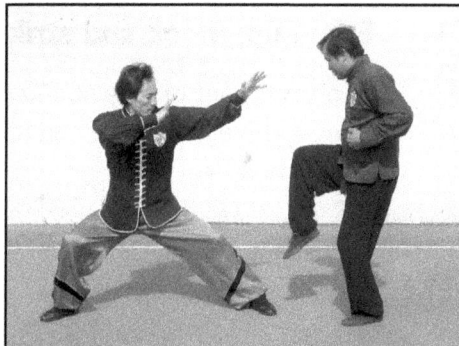

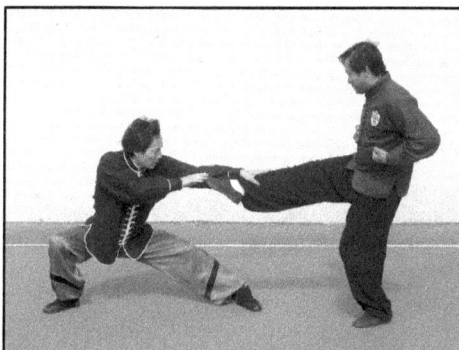

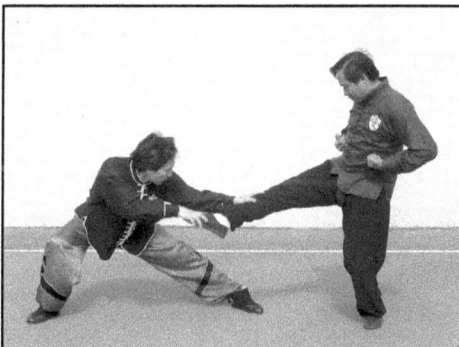

8A - Stand up. Block and strike.

Run towards your opponent and slap his strikes down with your hands. Leap up to kick him with your right leg.

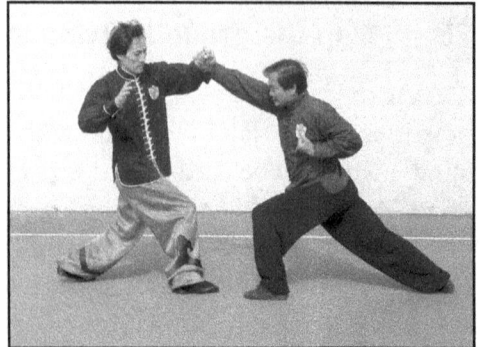

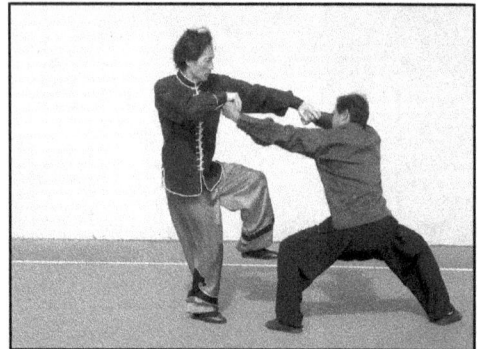

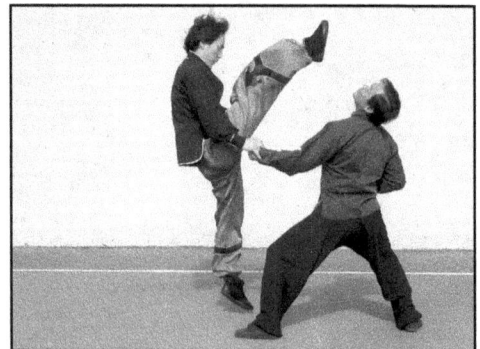

8B - Stand up. Block and strike.

If the kick fails to strike him, step forward, block upward with your left hand and strike him with the right fist.

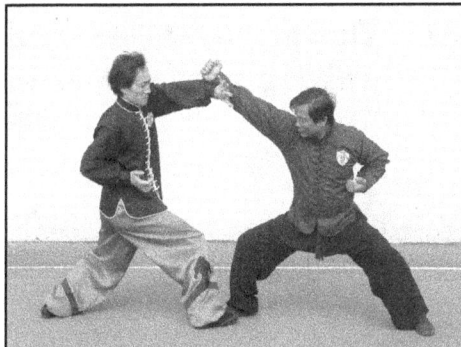

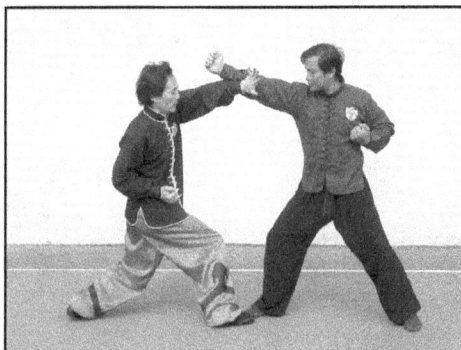

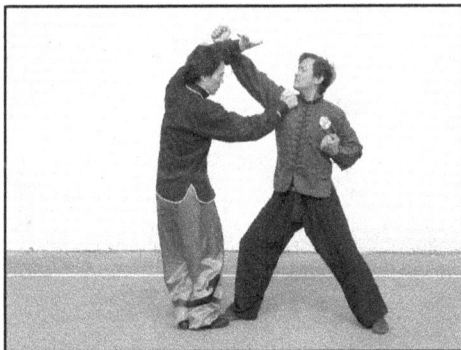

9 - Turn around. Willow tree swaying in the blowing wind. Go through the heart elbow. ("Protect the heart" elbow).

Clear his strike away with your left hand and use the right elbow to counterattack.

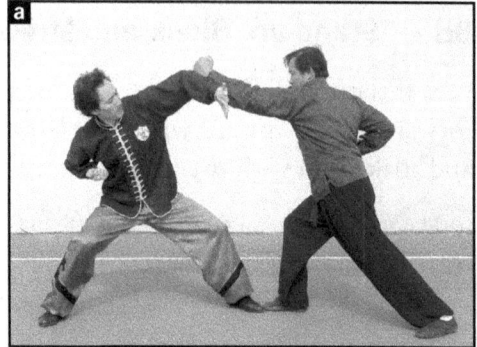

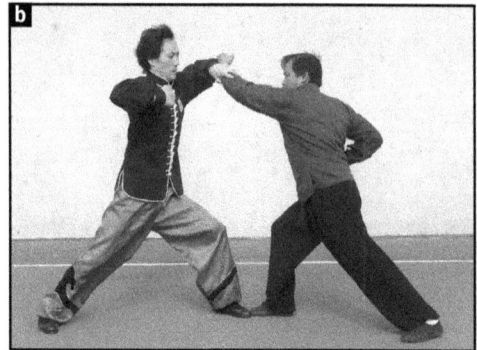

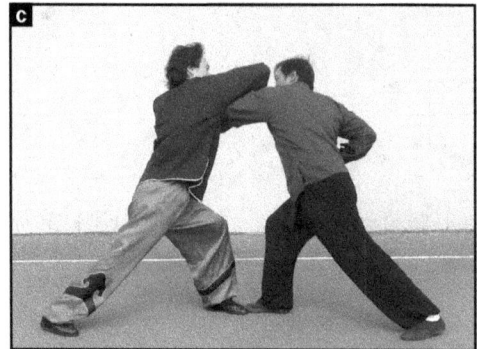

10A - Strike with the fist. (Backfist strike).

Parry his strike with your left hand and strike downward with the back of your right fist.

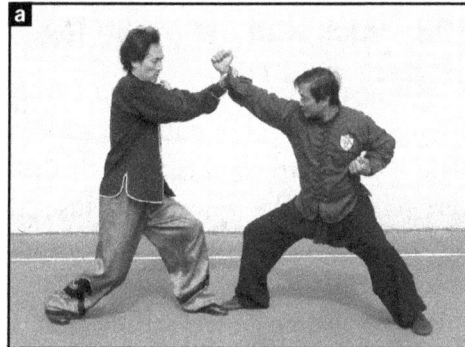

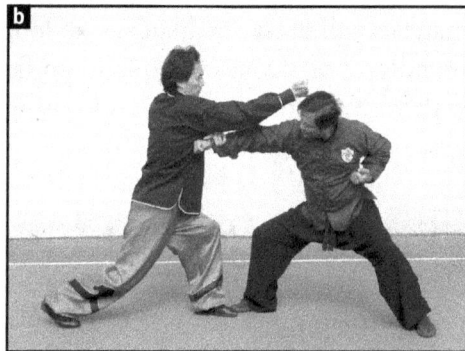

10B - Kick with the (right) leg.

If he grabs your right hand tightly and attempts to control or pull you, slide your right leg forward and kick him. If the kick is very powerful, this will surely cause "thunder down under." Only use this type of move in extreme situations with unsavory characters involving matters of real self-defense. Using movements such as these in friendly sparring matches will make the matches no longer friendly. Should you wish to remain friends with your sparring partner, avoid using such a technique.

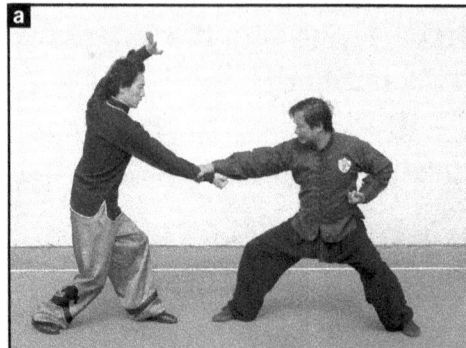

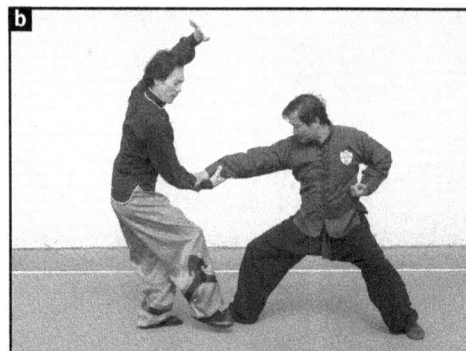

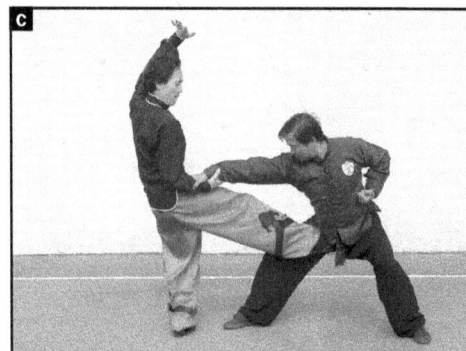

10C - Forward stance. Block and strike. (Right fist).

This again is a very basic motion. Block upward with your left hand and strike him with the right.

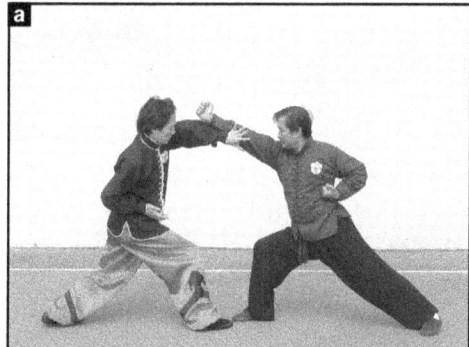

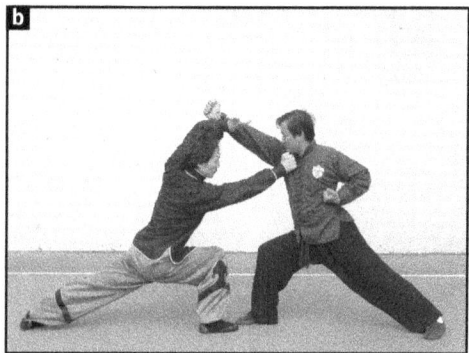

11 - Step forward. Uppercut palm strike to the groin.

As the name of the movement implies, raise his strike upward and strike with the fingertips of your left hand. You may strike him under the chin (as shown) or towards his throat.

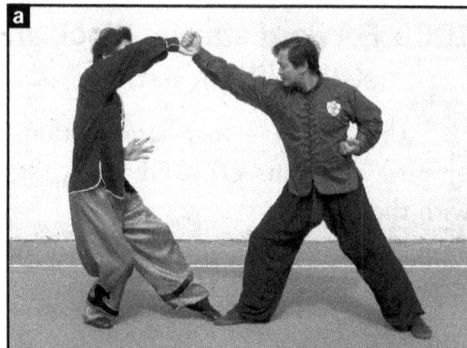

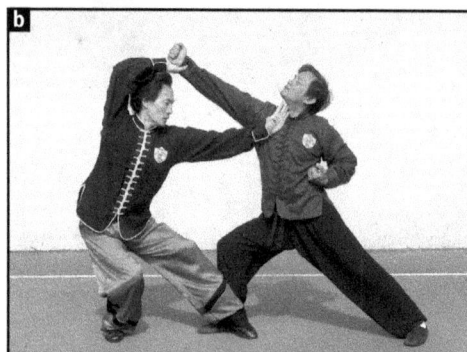

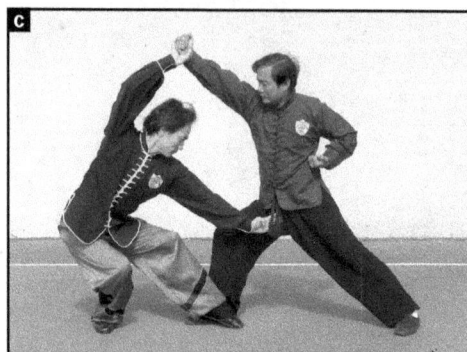

Or alternately, you may wish to cause fire down below.

12 - Stamp the ground. Strike with the fist.

Grab his left arm with your left hand, twist his arm using a counterclockwise motion, and strike him with your right fist. Simultaneously, you may stamp down on his left foot with your own right foot.

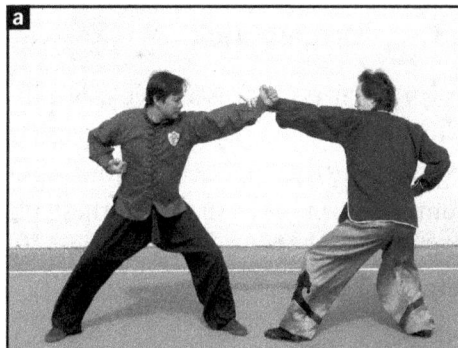

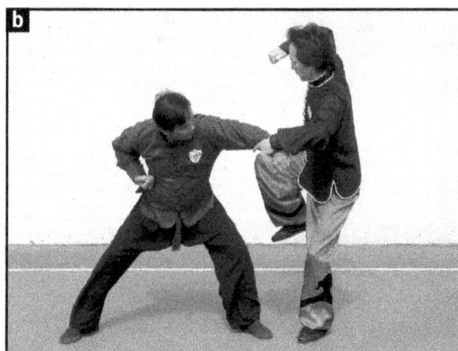

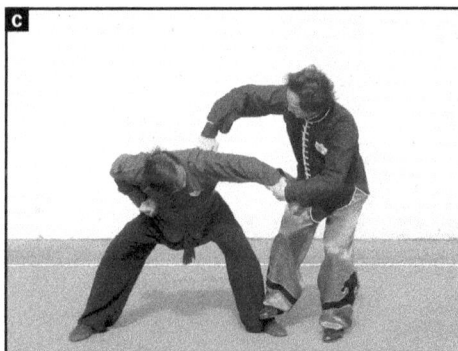

13 -   Tornado kick.

A tornado kick is a basic move in the Northern Shaolin Style. You may use the right leg to strike the opponent as your right leg is coming down, or as shown in these photos, you may use your right leg to strike the opponent in the face as your right leg is going up.

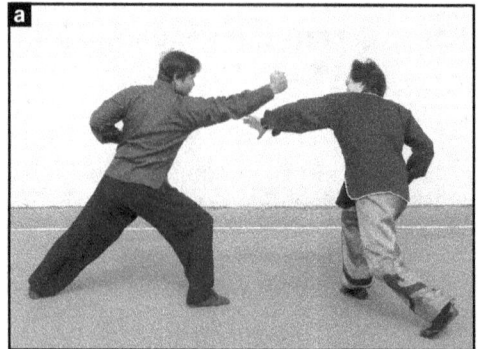

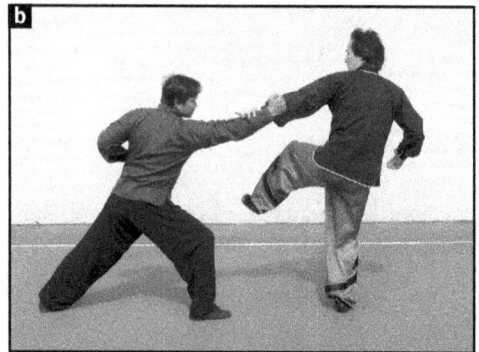

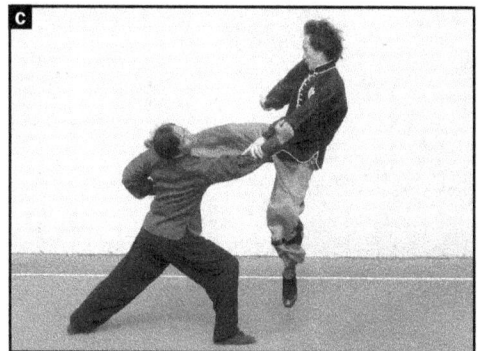

14 -   Goddess sprinkles the flowers.

Parry his strike downward with both of your hands, and then strike him in the face with the outer edge of your right hand.

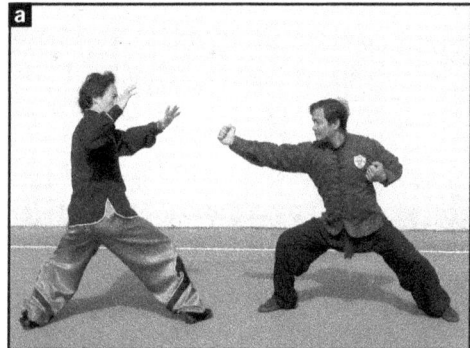

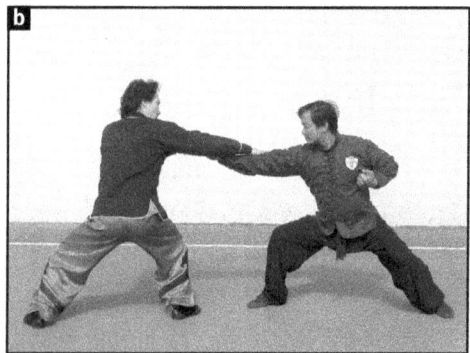

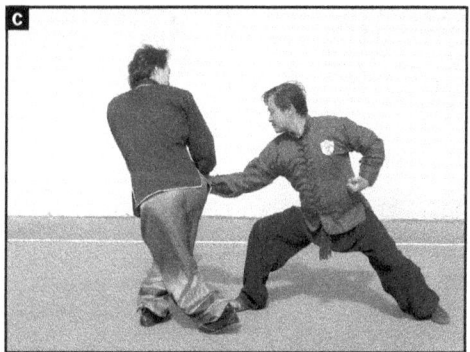

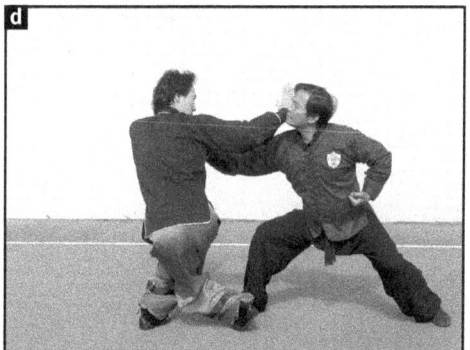

15A - Green dragon turns the body. (Right palm strike).

This is an advanced move. As my opponent rushes in to attack me, I twist my body around, thus removing his target area. I grab his left fist strike with my left hand and use a thrusting right palm strike to his head.

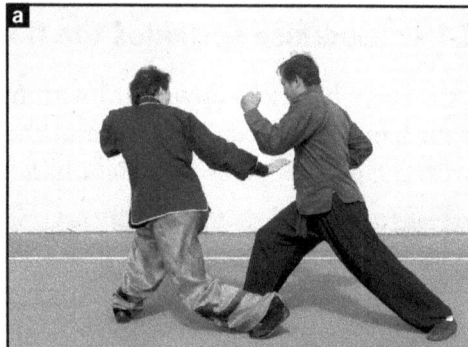

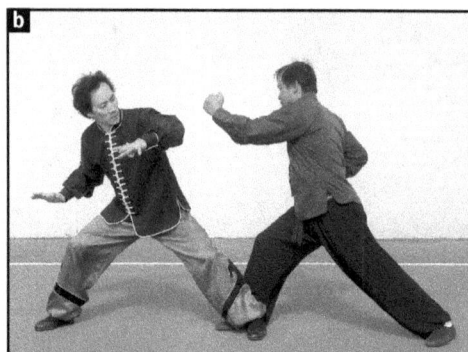

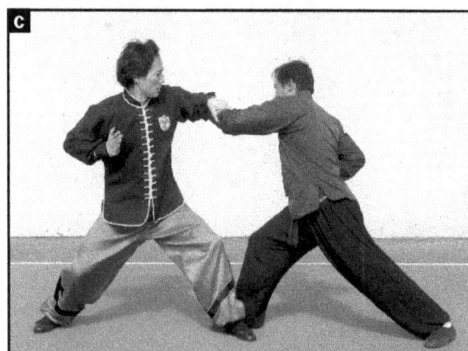

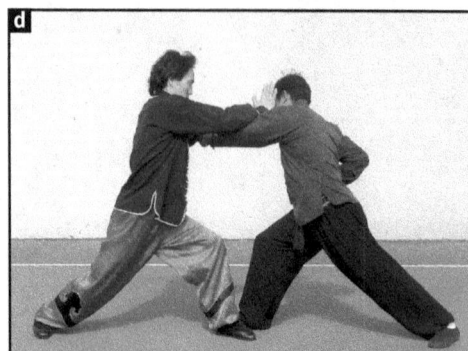

15B - Sit in a horse stance. Block and strike. (Left fist).

As my opponent strikes me with his right hand, I lift his arm and strike with my left fist.

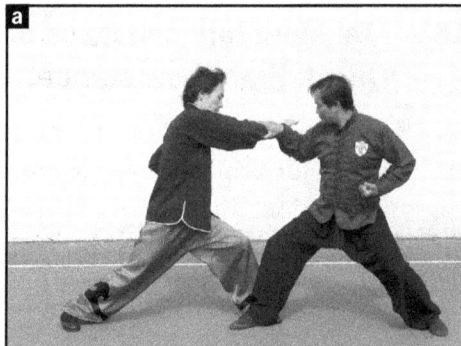

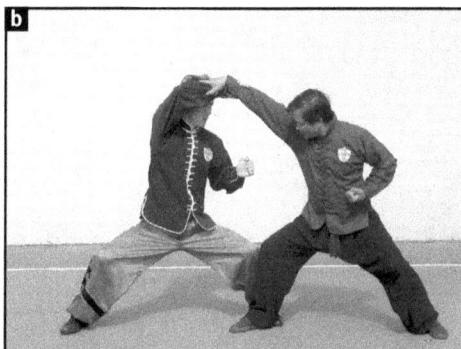

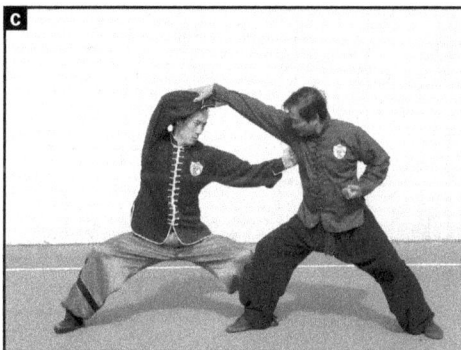

16 - Tai Mountain collapses on the head. Right bow stance.

As my opponent strikes with his left fist, I catch his left forearm and twist it in a counter-clockwise motion. Then I strike at the back of his left elbow with a right backfist.

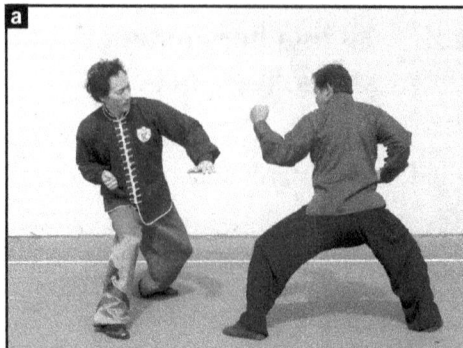

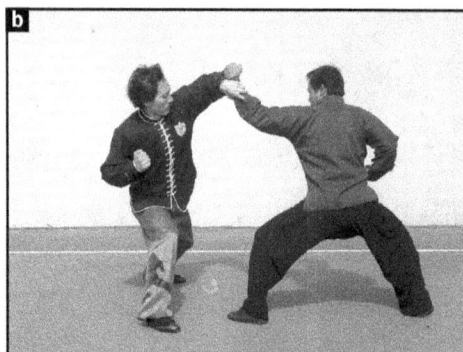

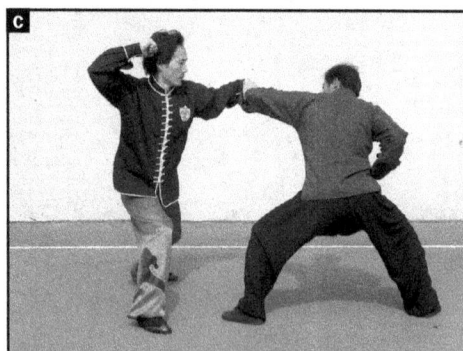

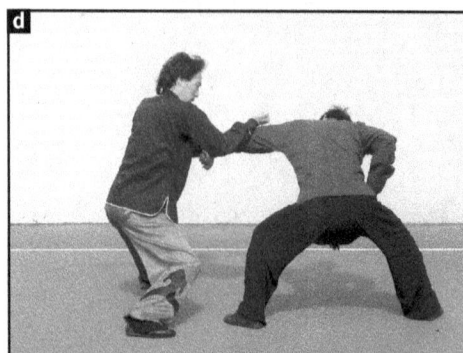

17A - Continuous flying kick.

This is another very basic motion in the Northern Shaolin Style. If he blocks your left kick, leap up and kick him with your right foot.

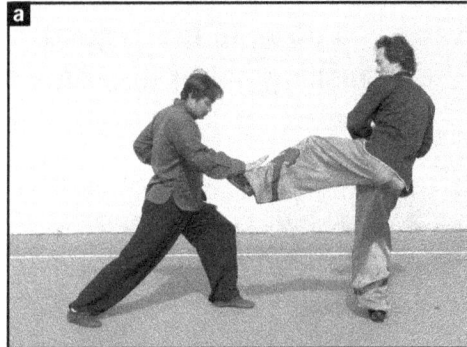

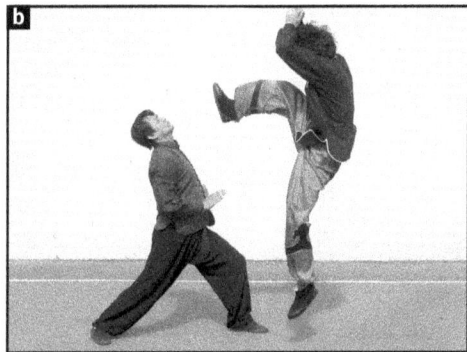

17B - Fall down to the ground. Double pushing palms in a right bow stance

If your opponent attempts to grab you, remove his hands from you by parrying up and outward with both hands, and then push forward forcefully at his chest. This two-handed motion is also very common in the style.

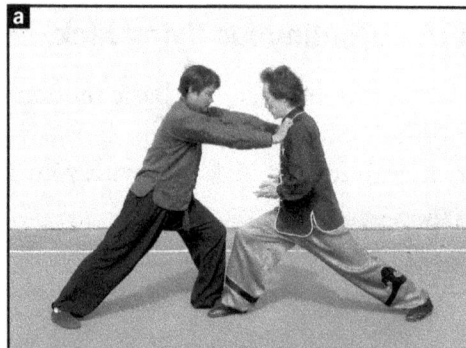

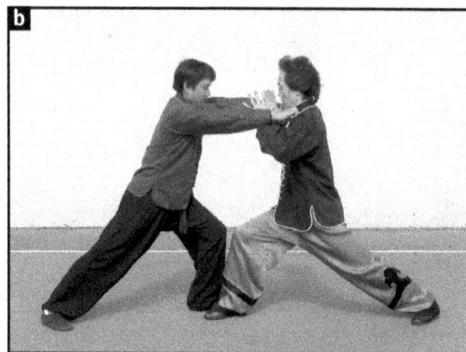

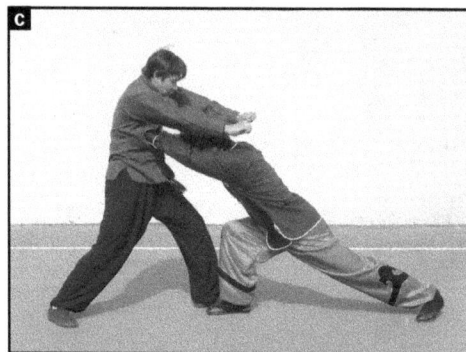

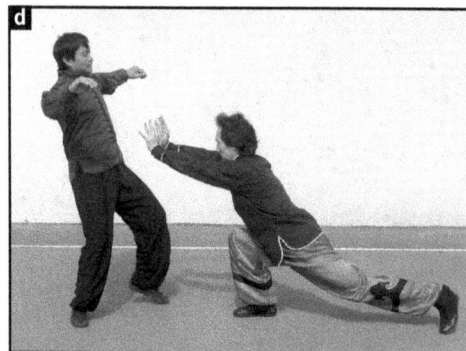

18A - Back sweep.

As before, as he attempts to strike
you high, move in and attack him low.
Sweep his forward leg so that he falls
down to the ground.

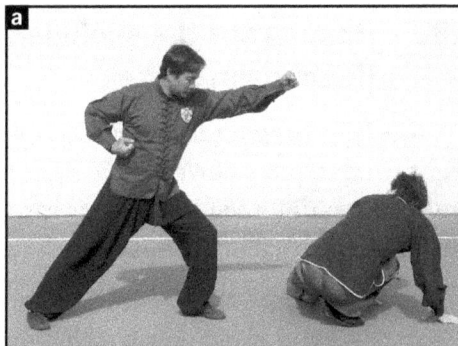

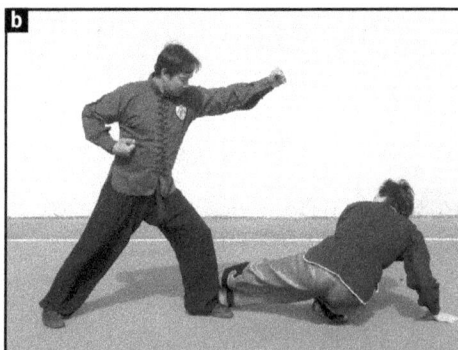

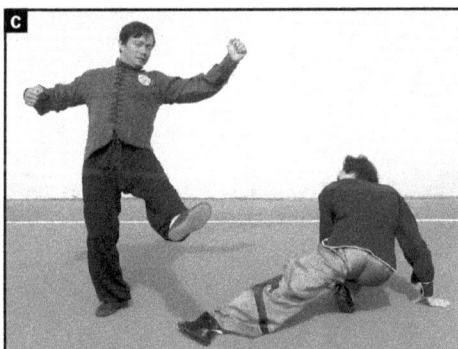

18B - Hawk grabs the shoulder.
(Right palm strike).

As he grabs your left shoulder, use your right hand to press down on his right hand to immobilize him, then swing your left forearm down on the back of his right elbow to turn him. Finally, strike him with your right hand.

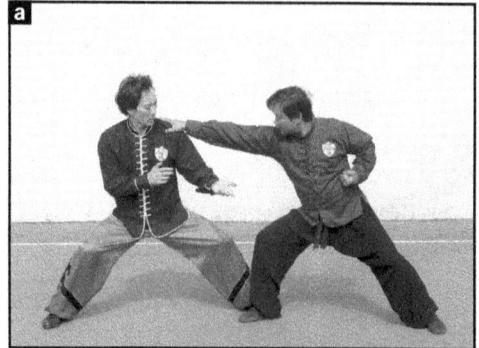

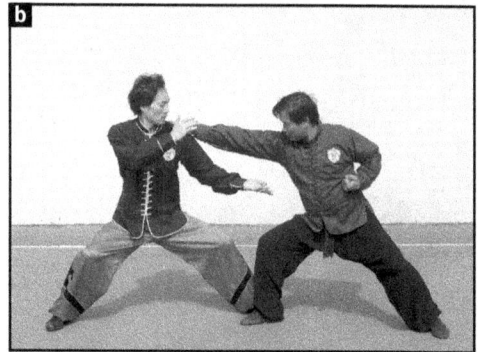

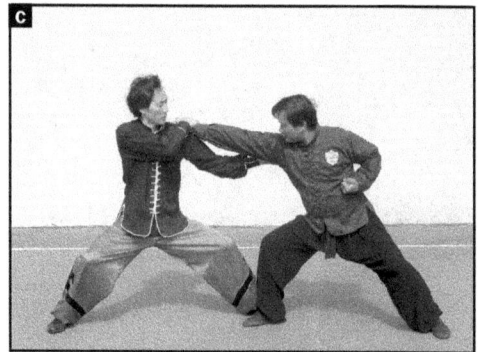

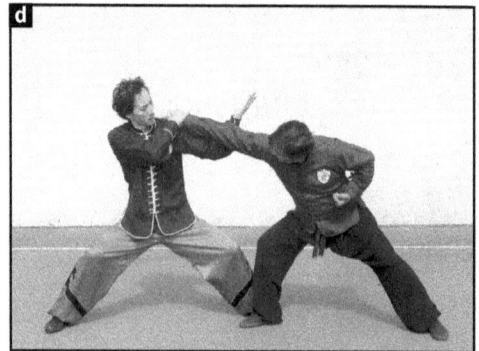

18B continued.

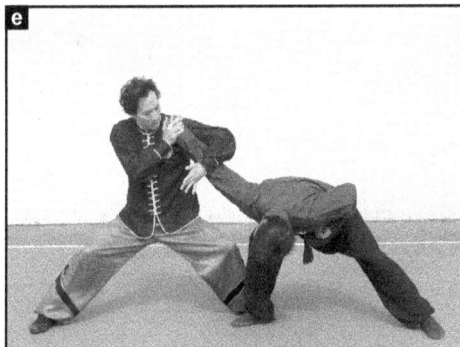

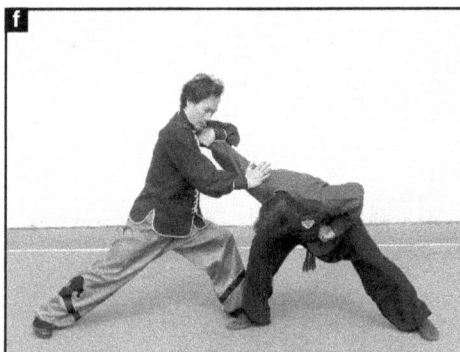

18C - Block and strike. (Left fist strike).

This is another basic motion of the "clear and strike" variety.

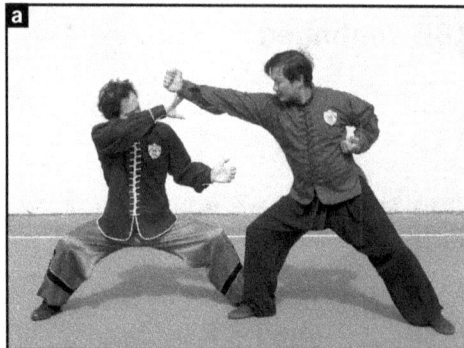

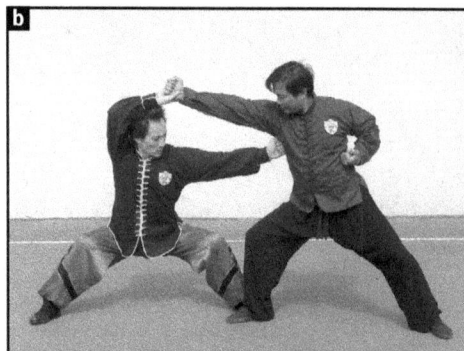

For movement #19 I shall give alternative applications. Multiple applications show the richness of the martial movements depicted in the forms. As you gain more experience, you will find more applications for the same move.

19 alternate A - Left and right, flip the hands upward.

As your opponent kicks with his left leg, step out to your right and scoop up his kick with the crook of your right arm. You now have the advantage as your opponent stands only on a single leg.

You may now sweep his leg out from under him. You may also raise his leg higher to make him fall.

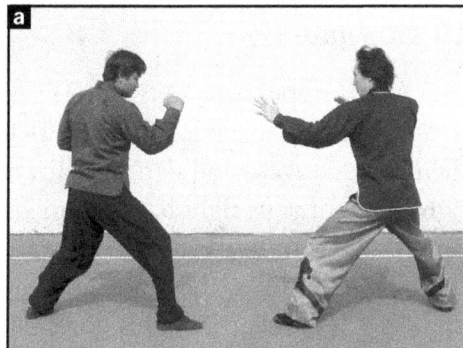

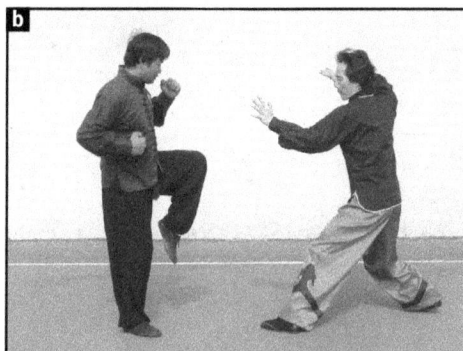

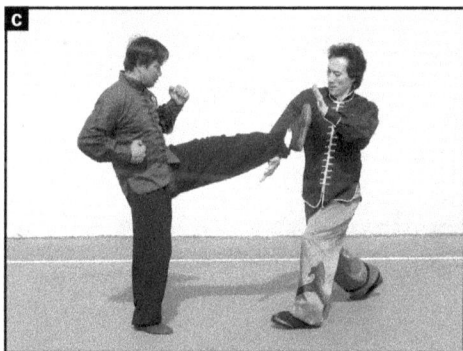

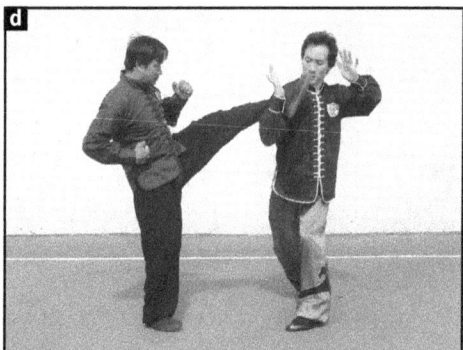

19 alternate B

As your opponent kicks with his left leg, rotate your body back to avoid the kick, and then come forward and slap the back of his right leg with your right hand to unbalance him. If you can time your slap so that you hit the back of his leg at the same moment the opponent is concentrating his power at the apex of his kick, so much the better.

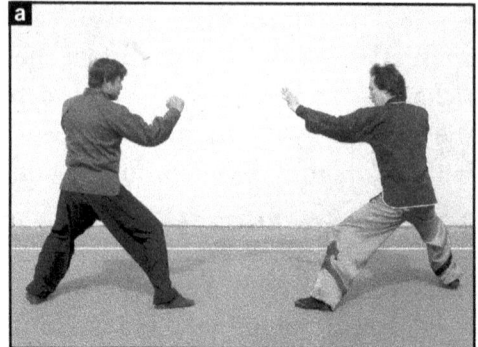

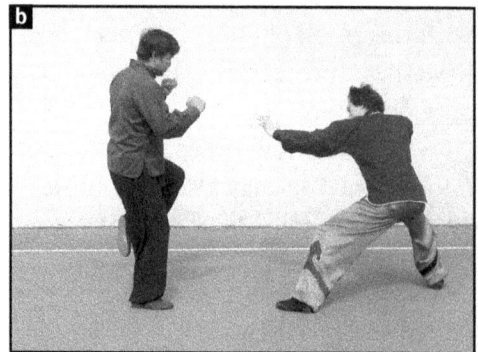

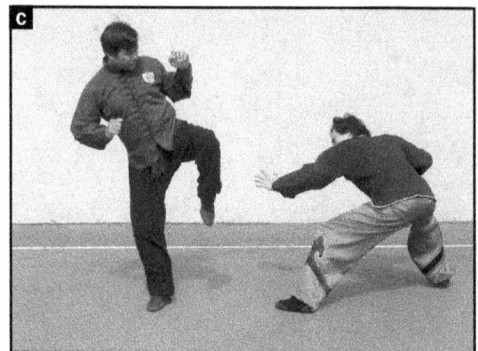

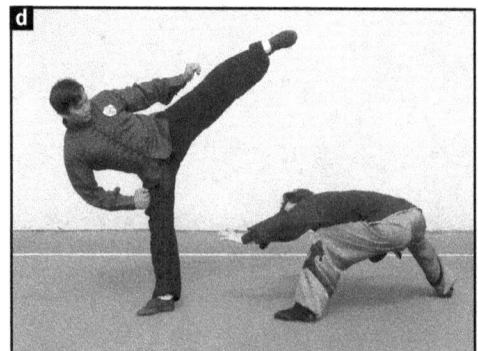

19 alternate B continued

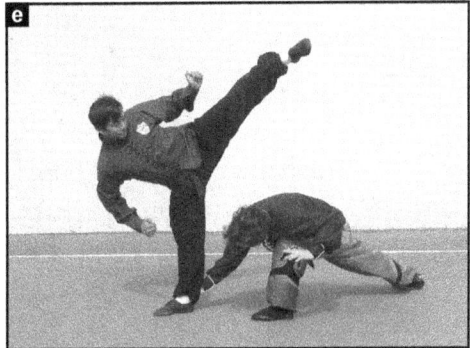

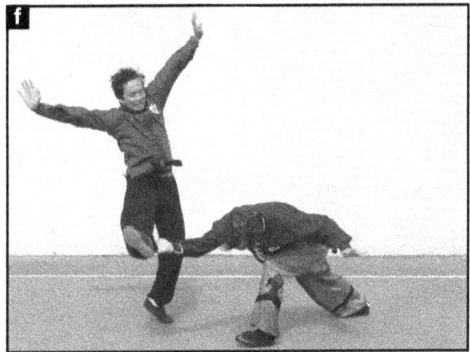

19 alternate C

Some practitioners will see the application with the raised knee as the main one. As the opponent strikes with his left hand, raise his left hand up and strike upward with your right knee to his midsection.

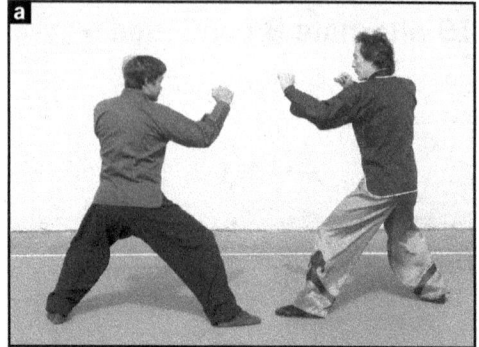

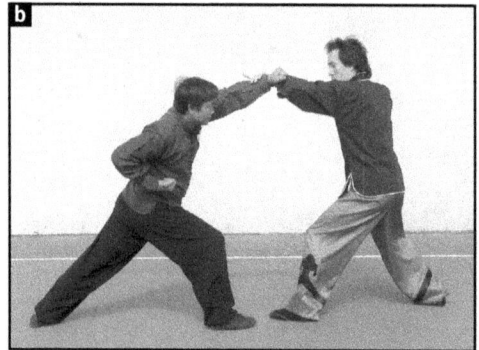

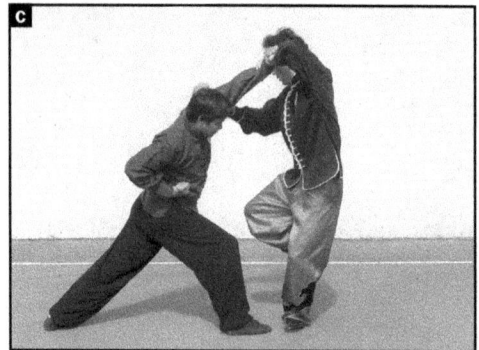

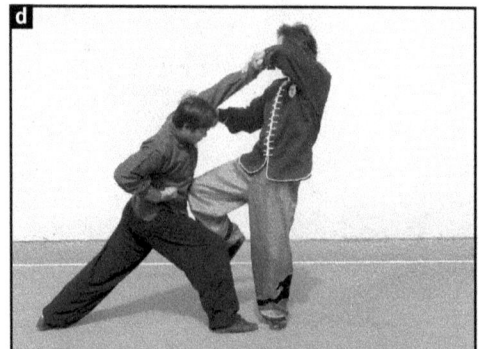

20 - Turn around. Right leg flying lotus kick.

Brush his attack aside with a sweeping motion of both of your arms, and if he retreats, jump forward and attempt to strike him with your flying lotus kick. Here the kick is performed as a forward lotus kick, but in the form it is performed behind you. The set teaches that a practicioner should be able to use their kick in any direction.

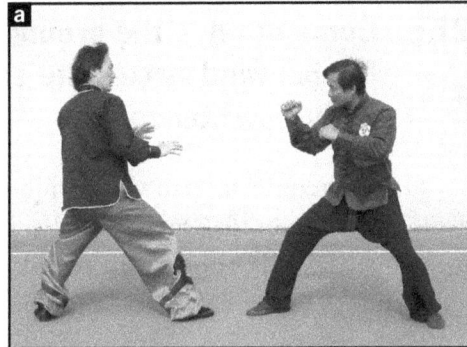

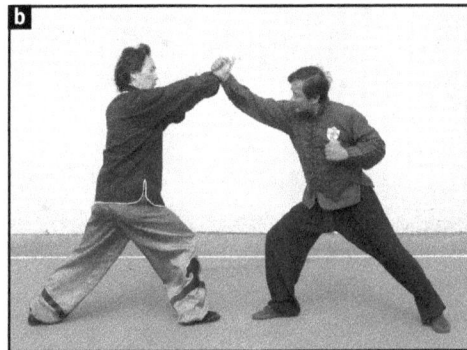

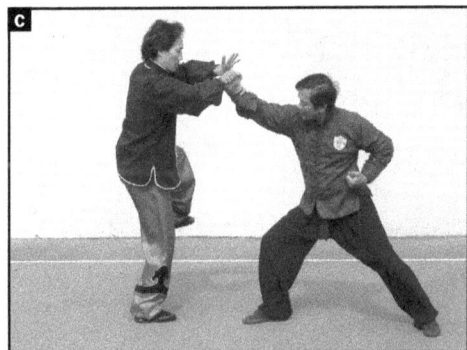

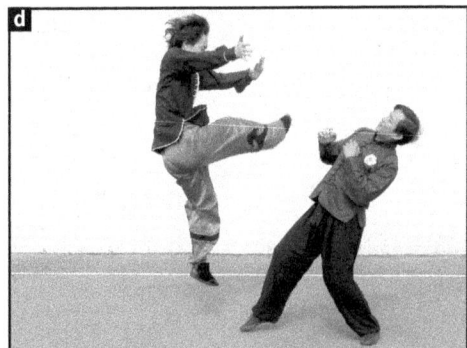

133

21 - Come down to the ground. Double wind strikes the ears. Right bow stance.

If he attempts to grab you with both arms, slap both of his arms down using your forearms, and strike him in the temple with your knuckles of your left and right hands.

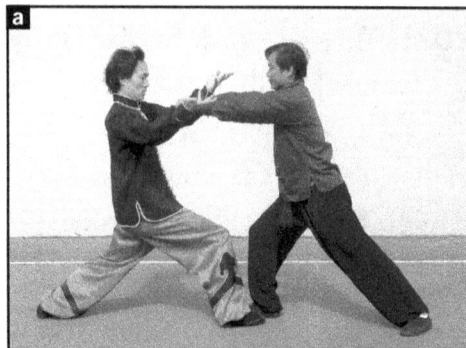

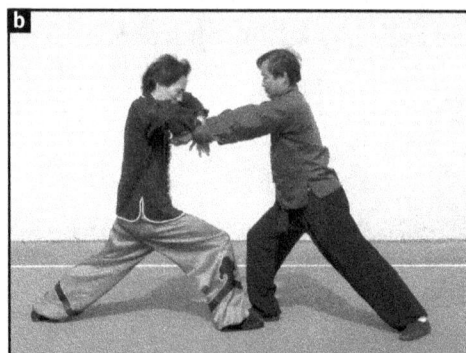

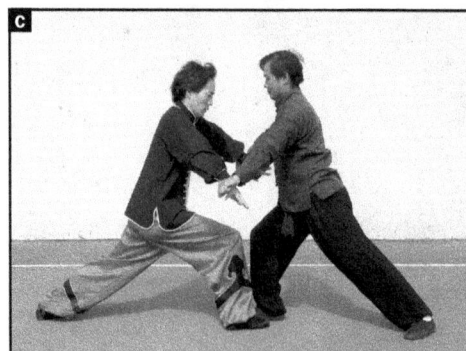

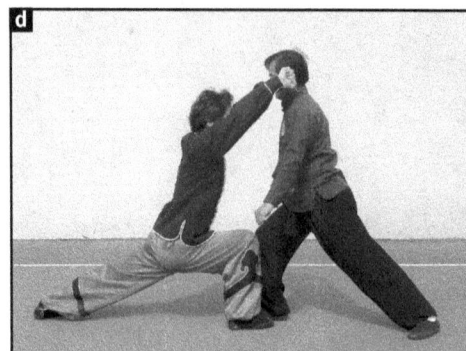

Continued on next page.

Movement #22 can be considered to have two parts.

22 alternate A - Twist stance. Thrust to the groin with both fists.

Kick forward with your left leg so that you hook his front leg and unbalance him.

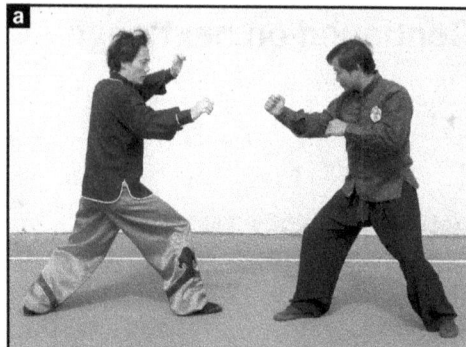

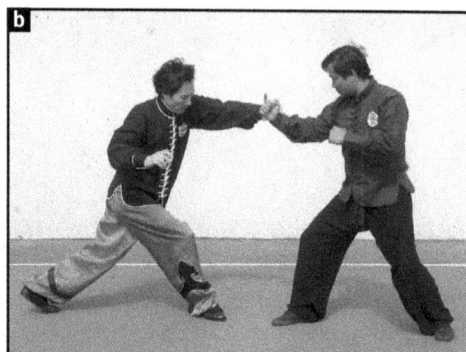

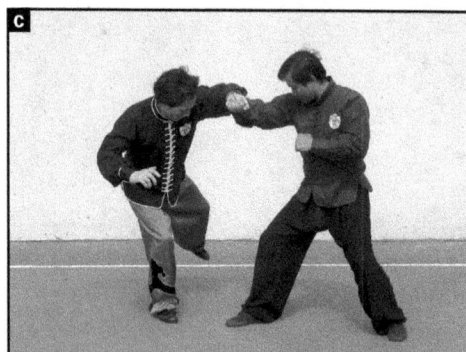

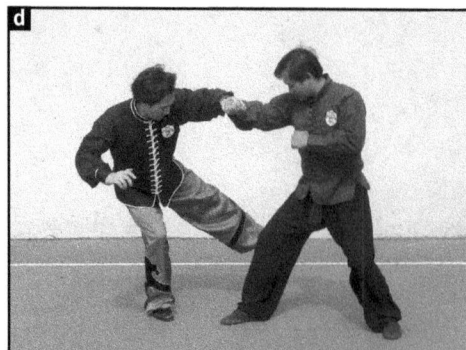

22A continued.

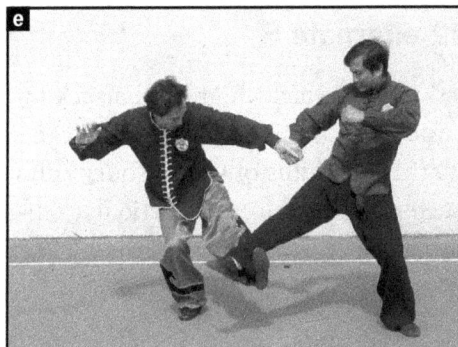

22 alternate B

As he attacks high, you attack low and punch him between his legs. We can safely say that the Marquis of Queensbury rules have been suspended in this particular self-defense situation.

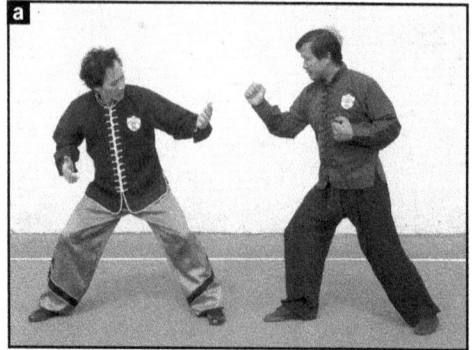

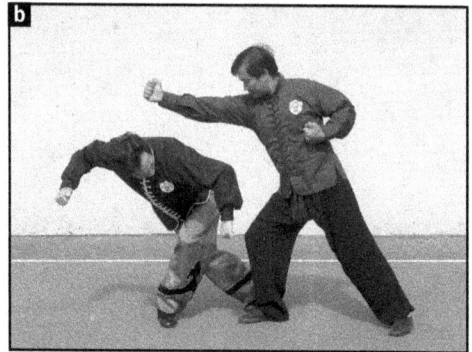

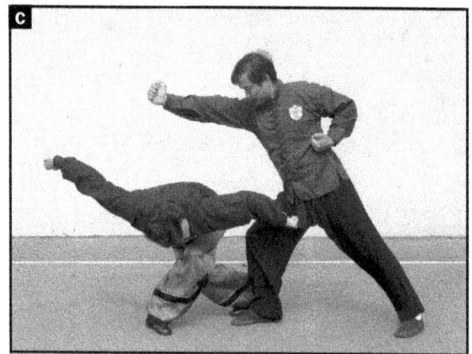

22 alternate C

Alternatively, as he punches high, you can grab him down below. I suppose this gives a whole new meaning to "reach out and touch someone."

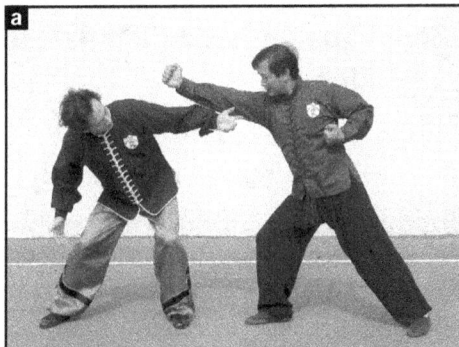

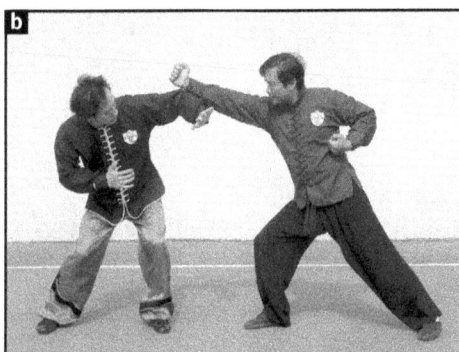

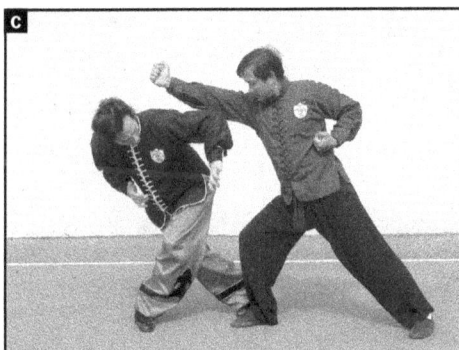

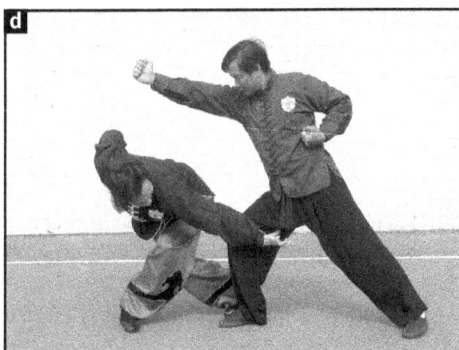

23A - Flipping hand (fist), left thrust kick.

This is another very basic motion, that of the side kick. Although the move is performed in the set using a left punch, you may use your left hand here not to strike the opponent, but instead to deflect his punch. Simultaneously, kick out with your left leg into his midsection.

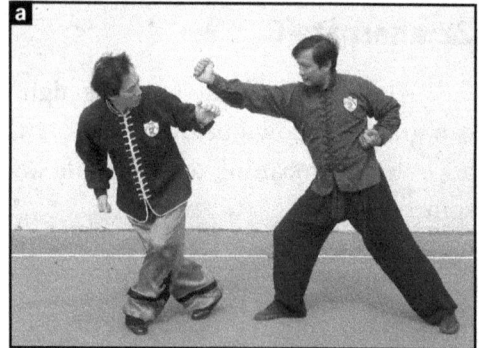

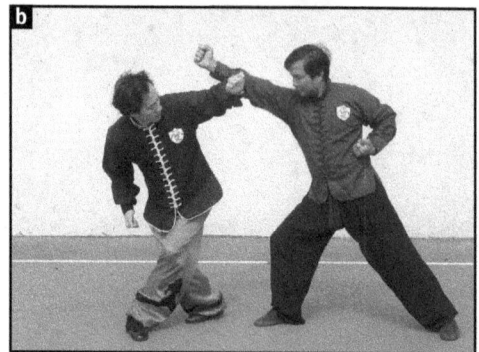

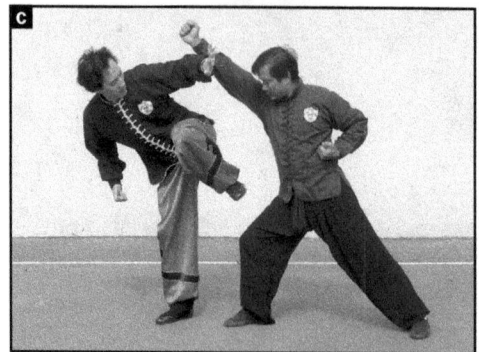

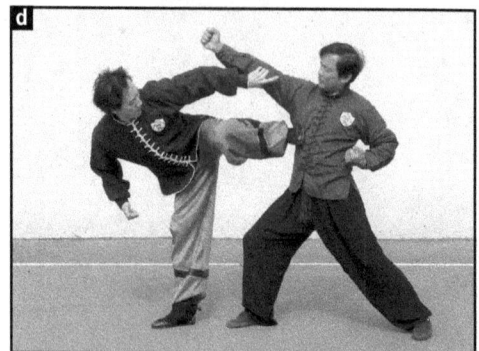

23A continued

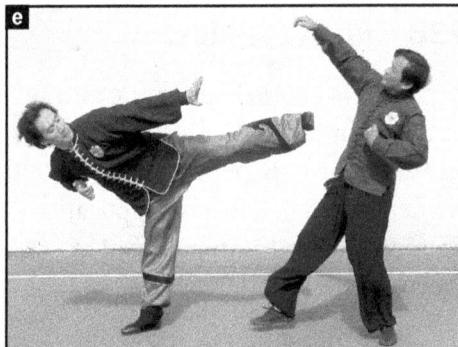

23B - Right toe kick.

This is another very basic motion, that of the front toe kick. This kick may be used to attack the opponent at any level, although we depict here a low-level application. As the opponent attempts to grab you or push you, kick upward with force.

This move will stop most opponents in their tracks, rather completely. If this doesn't stop your opponent, run away quickly.

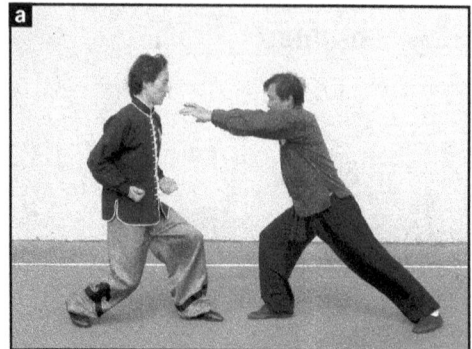

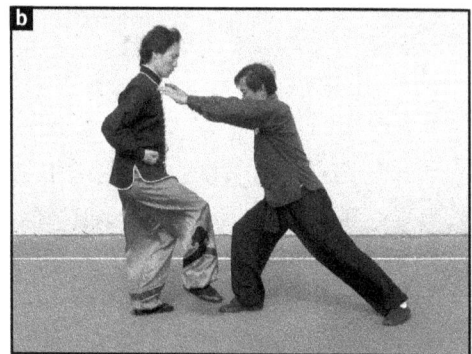

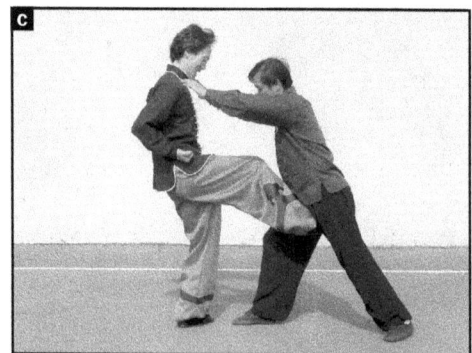

23C - Double pushing palm.

Here we have another very basic motion, that of pushing forward with both of your palms. As he attempts to push you, separate his arms, and return the favor by pushing back at him.

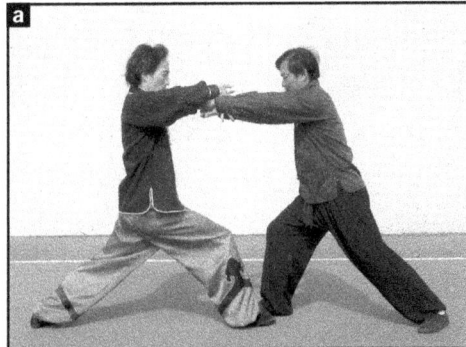

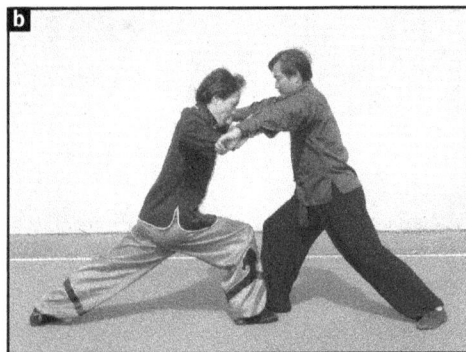

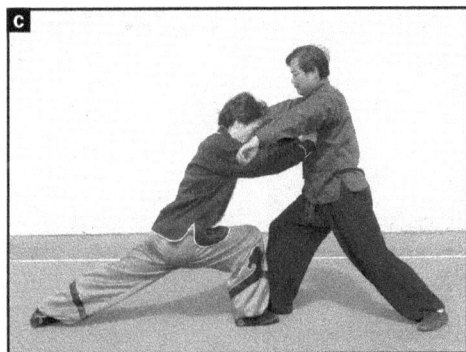

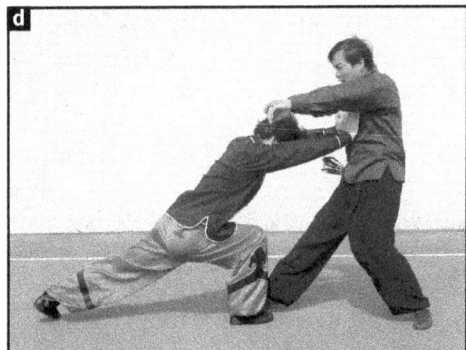

Only when you realize that your move is a "finishing" blow should you put your full force into it.

24 - Full back sweep.

We have shown the application of this movement before. Use your left leg to sweep your opponent's lead leg out from under him.

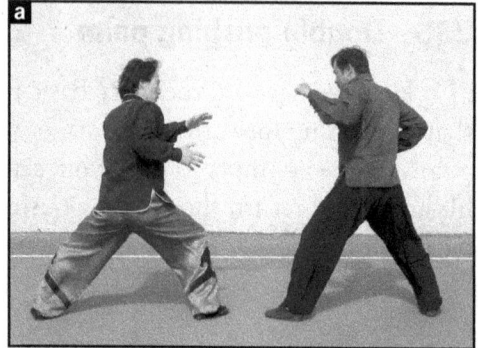

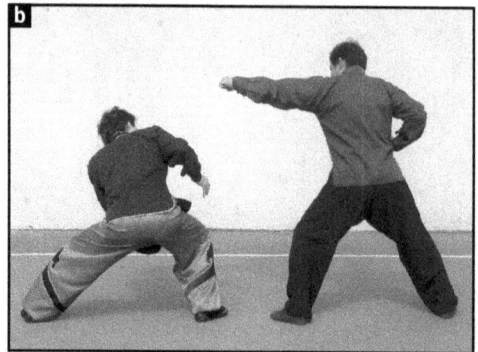

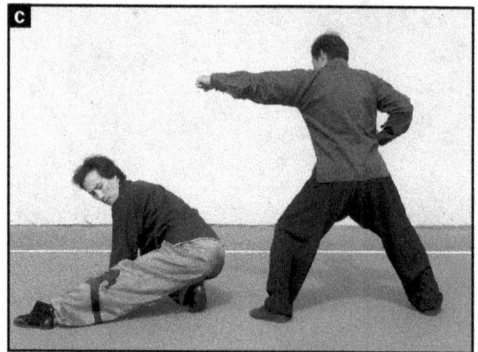

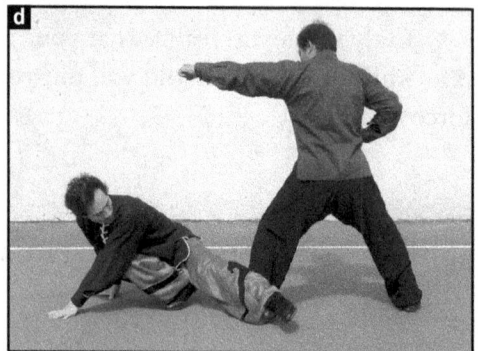

24 continued

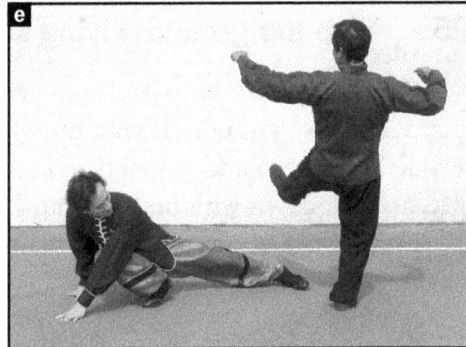

25 - Slap the ground. Flying sand.

You complete your sweep and are in a very vulnerable position. If your opponent has avoided the sweep and attempts to kick you, slap his kick down with both of your hands.

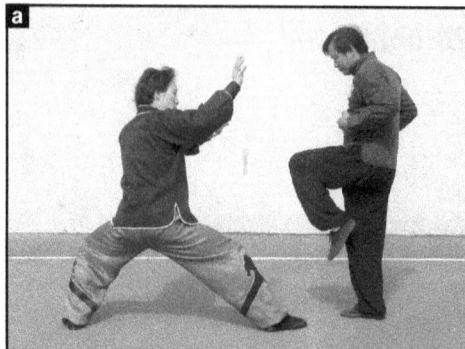

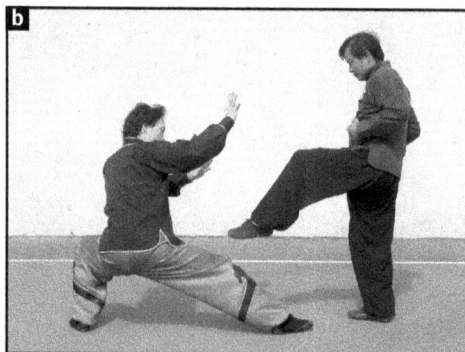

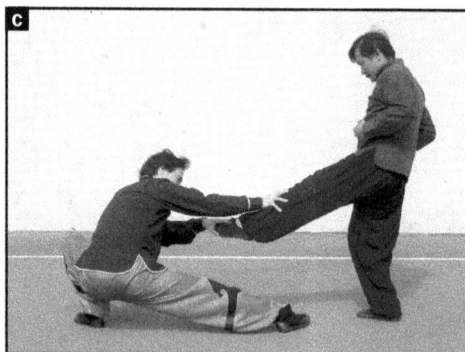

26 - Double kick.

The double kick is a very popular kick in the Northern Shaolin Style. Slap his strikes down, leap forward, and kick upward.

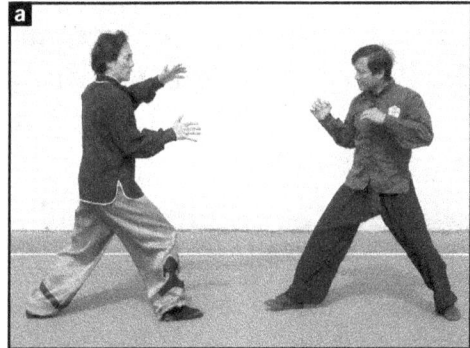

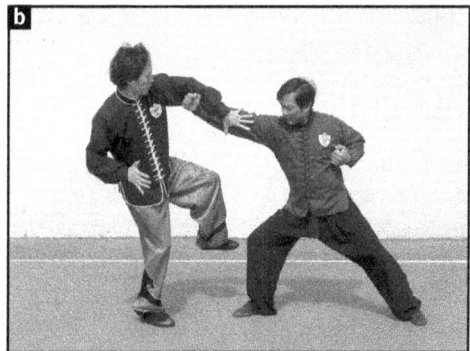

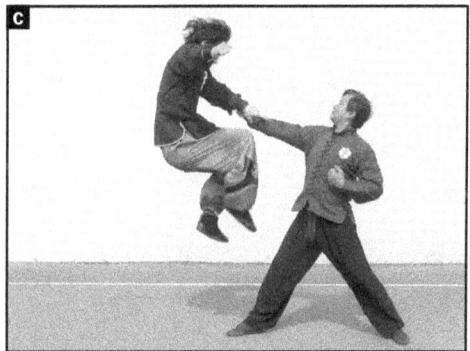

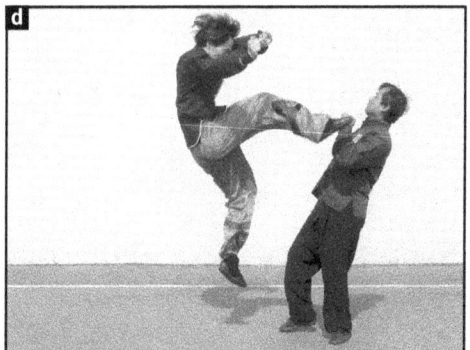

A deadly kick to the throat.

27 - Come down to the ground. Right bow stance. Block and strike. (Left blocks and right fist strikes).

Suppose he backs away and you cannot catch him with your double kick. As he punches you, raise his arm up and strike him with your fist. This is another typical application that falls under the general category of "clear and strike."

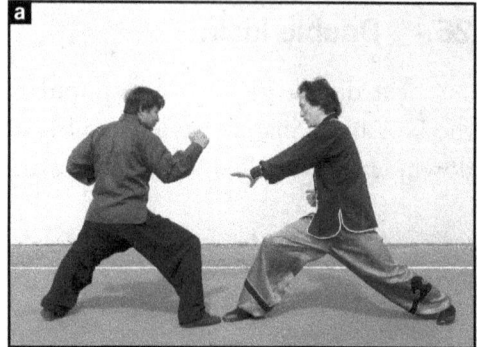

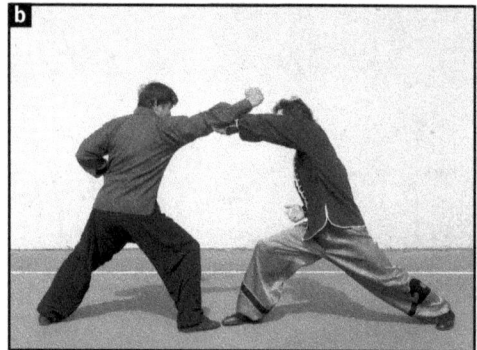

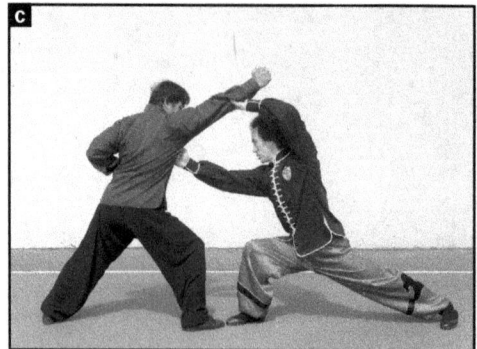

28 - Steal a step. Wipe off the hand. Block and strike.

Similar to the application as shown previously, clear his strike with your right hand, and strike him in the southern region with your left fist.

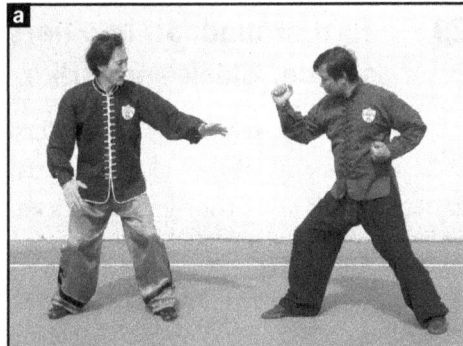

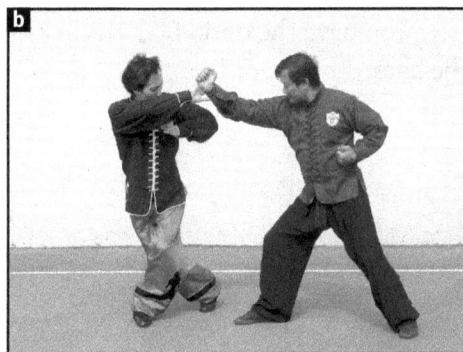

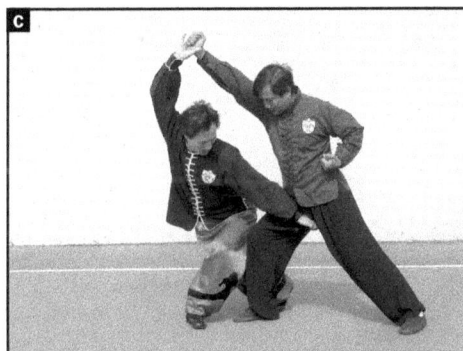

29 - Turn around. Sit in a horse stance. Block and strike.

By now, the reader should understand these movements of the "clear and strike" variety. Block with your left hand and strike with your right fist.

You have the option of striking him in the chest, throat, or face.

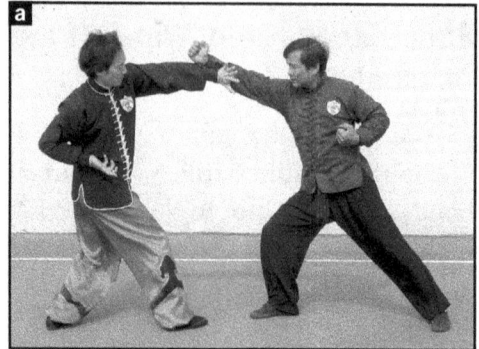

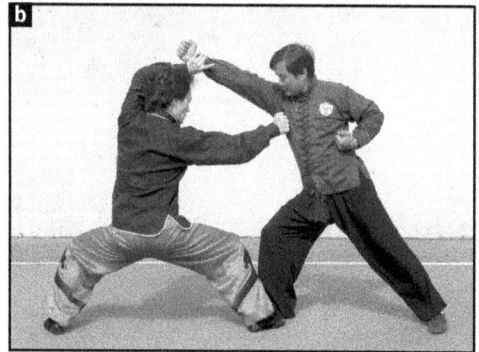

30A - Raise the right leg.

Carefully read your opponent's body motion, and as your opponent attempts to sweep you, lift your right leg.

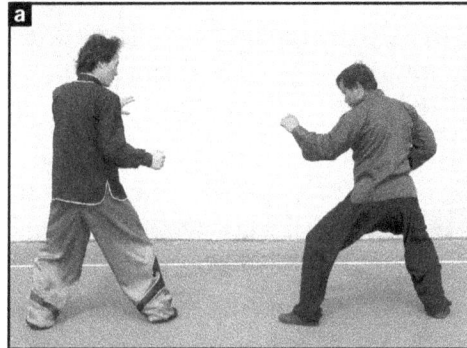

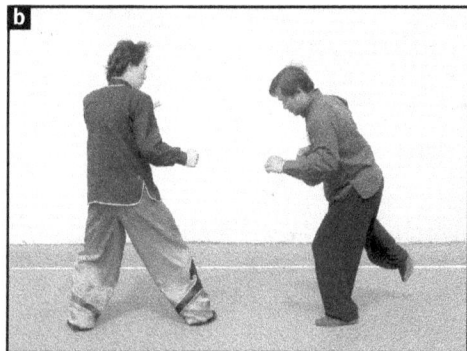

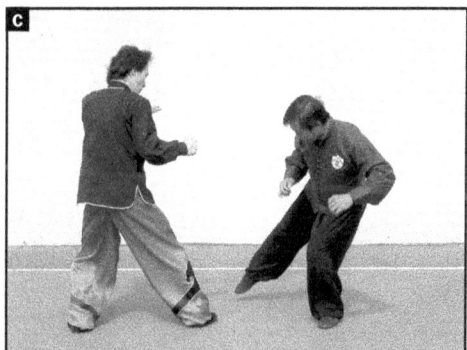

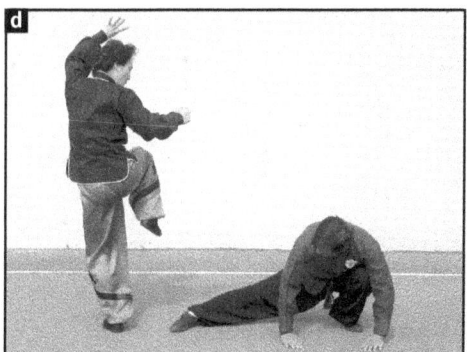

30B - Stamp the foot. Tangling hand. Step forward. Press and strike with the fist.

As he attempts to strike you, grab his right wrist with your right hand, pull him in and control him by using your left hand to grip his right forearm, and then punch him with your right fist.

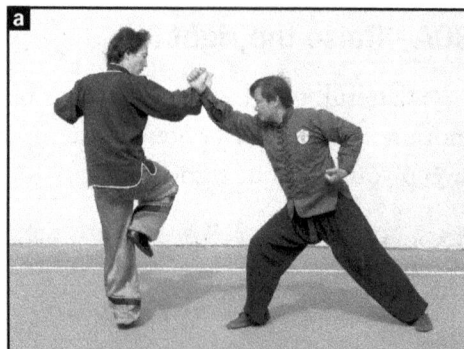

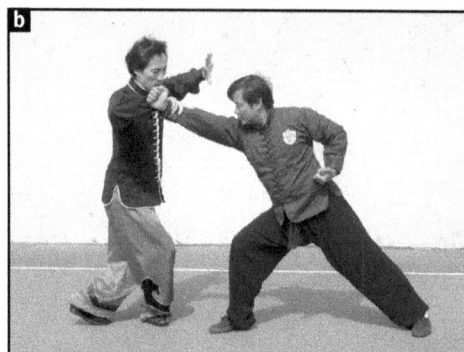

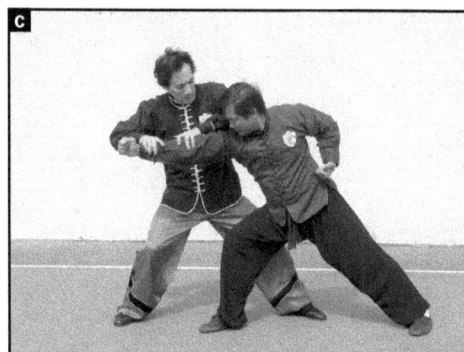

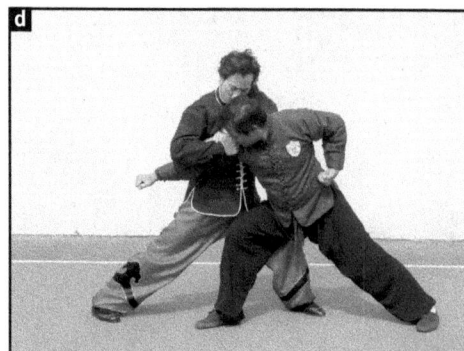

30B continued

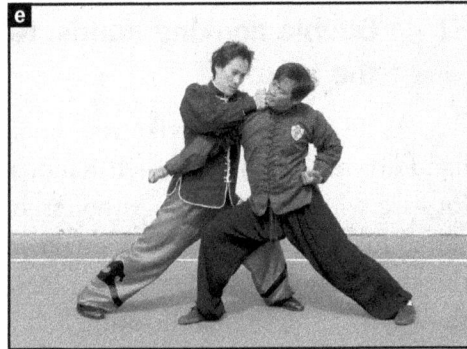

31 - Double hooking hands. Kick to the face.

As he attempts to strike you, hook his hand downward with your left hand, and kick forward with your left leg. Although in the actual form, both hands hook downward and the kick is done with the right leg, here we show only a single hand hooking and the left leg kicking. Applications as indicated by the form can be done on any side or with any arm or leg, depending on the situation.

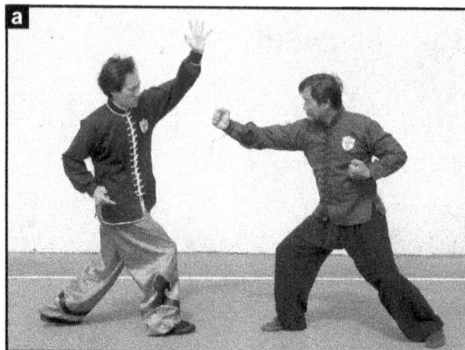

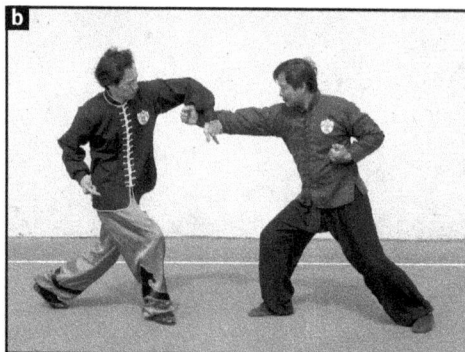

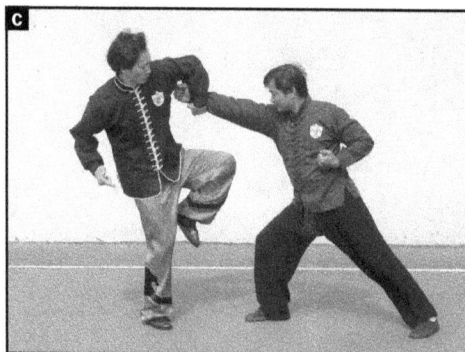

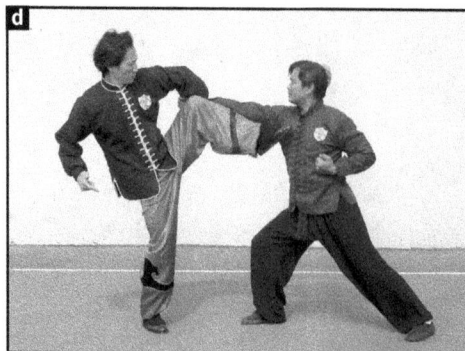

31 continued

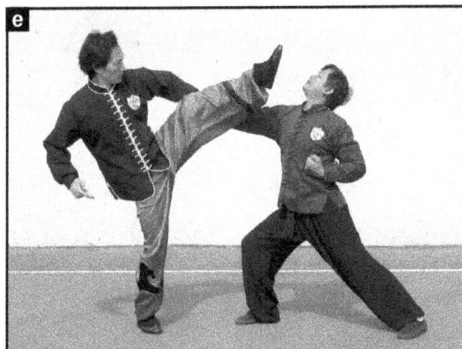

32A - Double uplifting hands.
Flying kick.

As the name of this move indicates, block upward with the hand and kick forward.

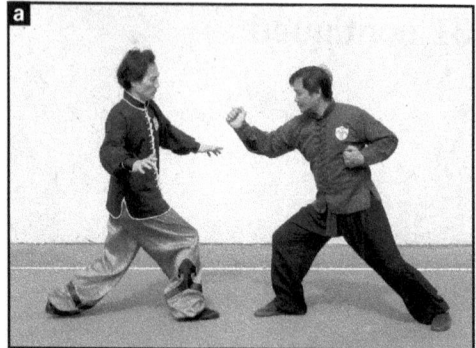

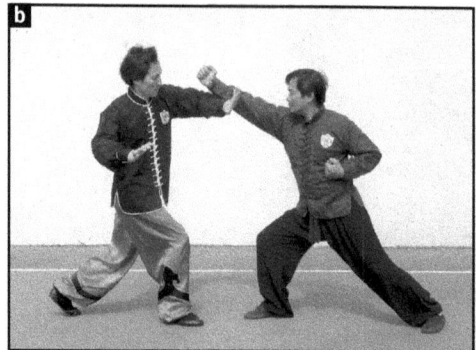

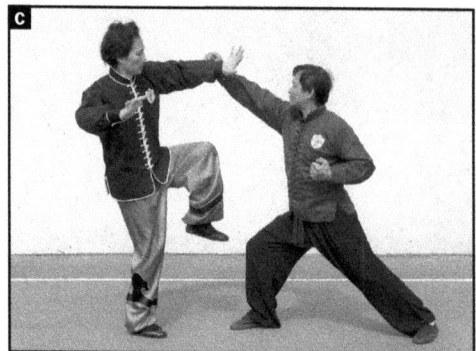

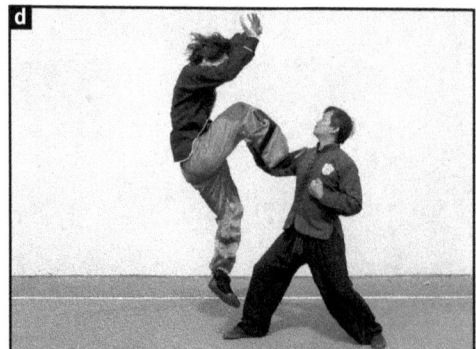

A reprise of the deadly double kick. This is a kick to the throat.

32B - Come down to the ground in a left bow stance. Double pushing palms.

This motion is another basic motion. Push forward with both palms to attack his chest. If he takes the outside, claim the inside for yourself.

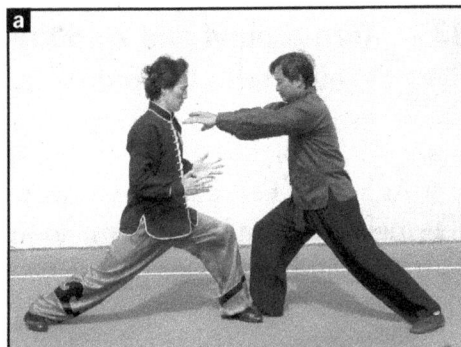

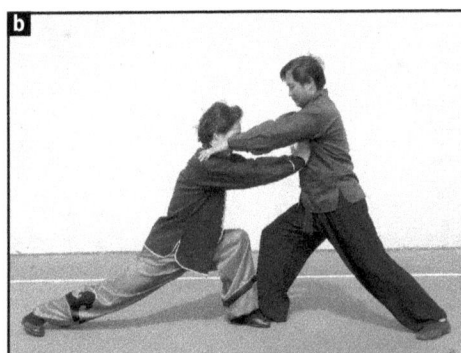

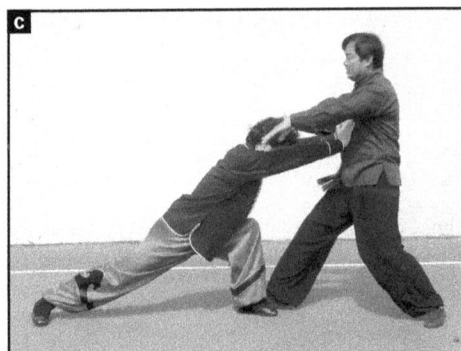

33 - Turn around and slap the ground with the palms in a cross-legged stance.

As he punches you, grab his wrist with your right hand, and press down on his elbow with your left hand. Force him down to the ground if possible.

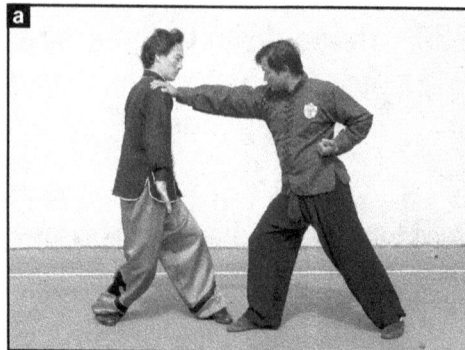

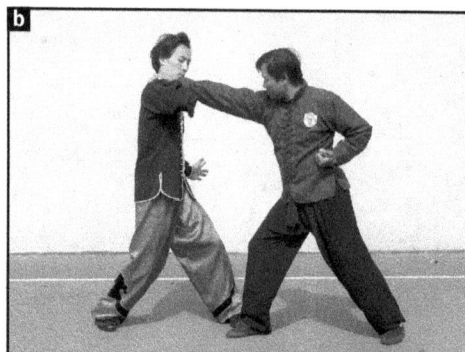

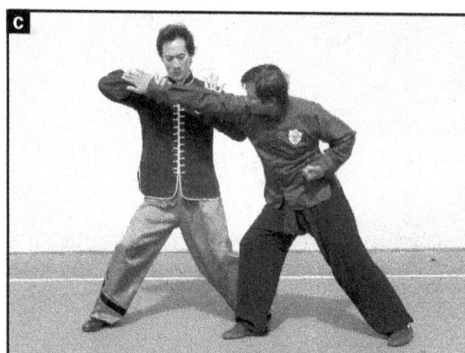

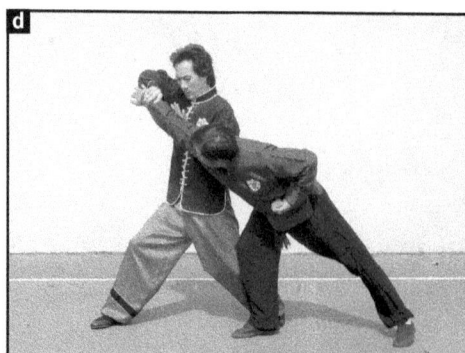

33 continued

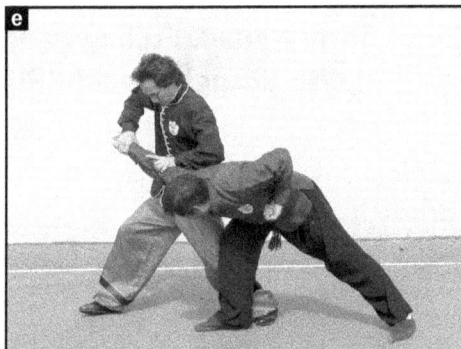

34 - Turn around. Pulling hand (Left). Straight punch (Right).

As the name of this movement implies, pull him in with your left hand and strike him with your right fist.

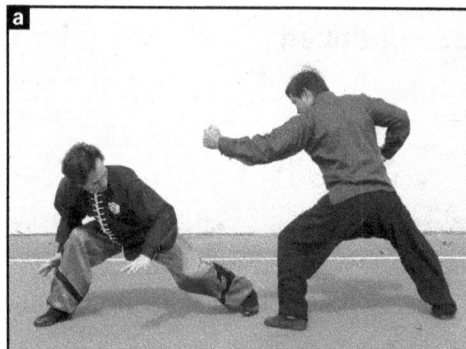

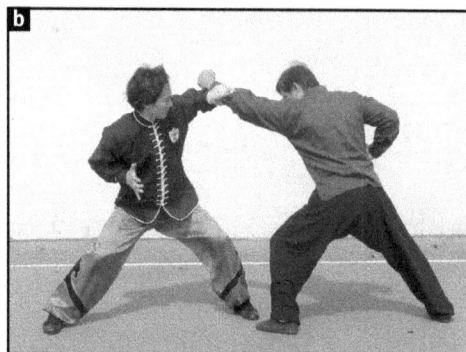

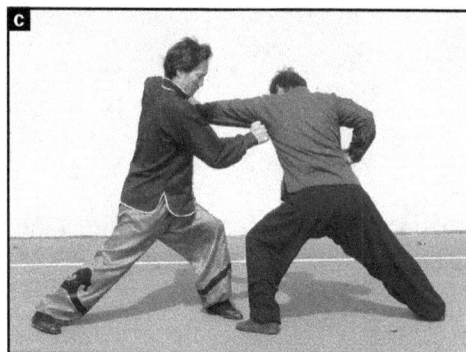

35 - Right kick.

This is another basic motion, that of the right thrust kick. Parry his strike with your left hand (even though in the set the movement is done as a fist strike), and kick forward with your right leg using the heel as the contact point.

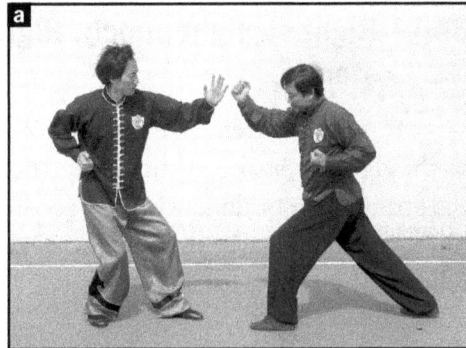

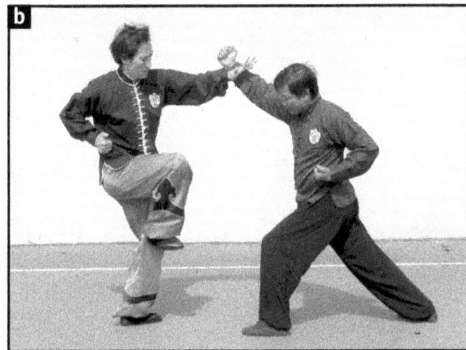

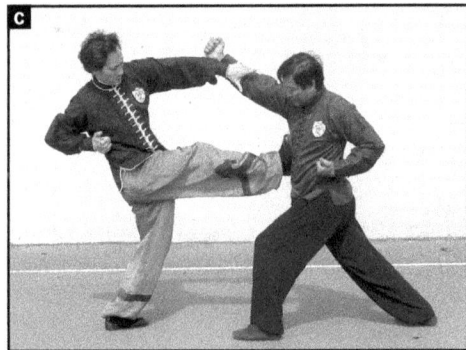

36A - Right straight punch. Right bow stance.

This is an extremely basic motion, that of the right fist strike. Although in the set the strikes are not done with a preceding block, the photos will show a left hand parry, followed by a right fist strike.

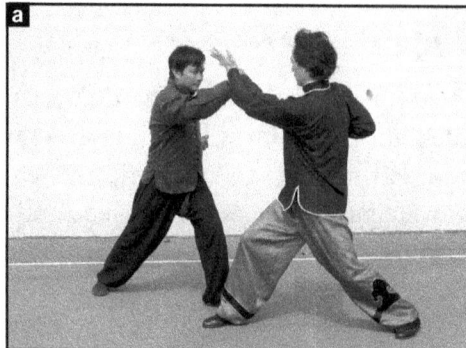

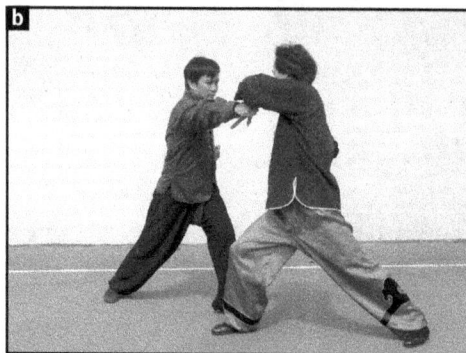

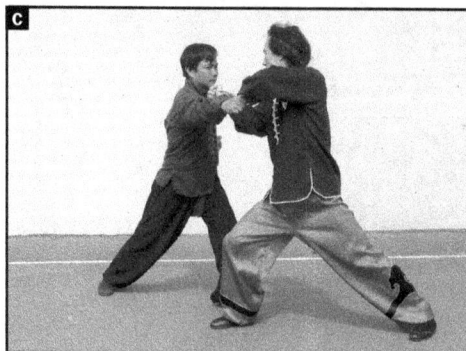

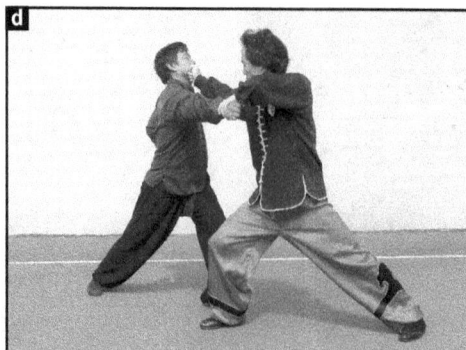

36B - Left straight punch. Right bow stance.

This is the same action as in 36A, except the fist strike is done with the left fist. In the photos, I clear with my right hand and strike with my left to defend against his left hand strike.

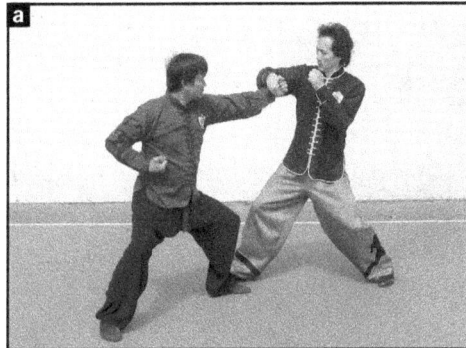

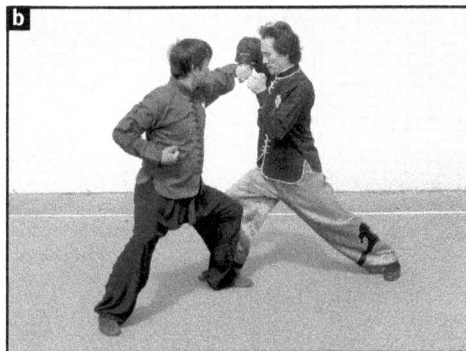

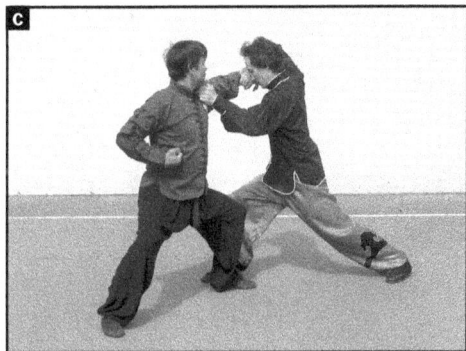

37 - Tornado kick.

The tornado kick is a kick that can be used as a defensive move from any position. Leap up and strike him in the head with your right foot. Time this movement so that torque and momentum are on your side.

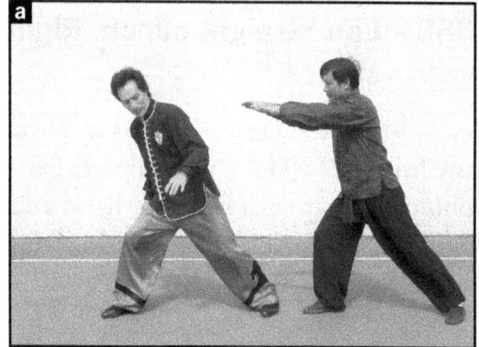

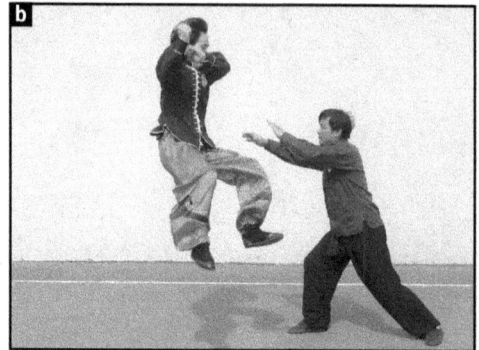

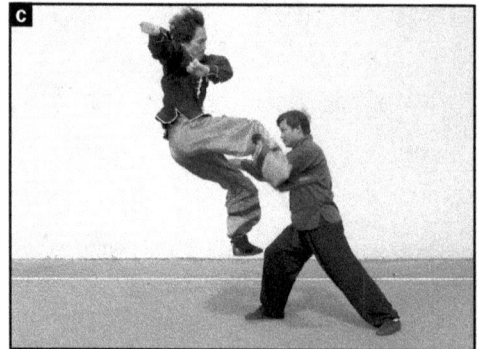

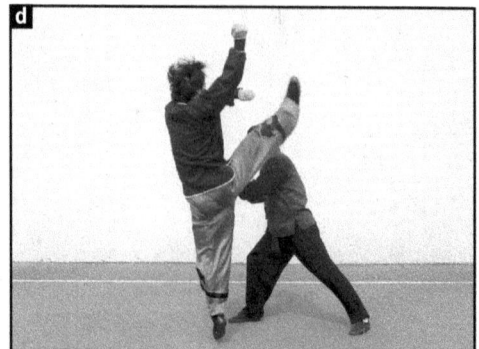

37 continued

You and your former opponent may now resume quiet, civilized, verbal discussion. The tornado kick was merely an interjection.

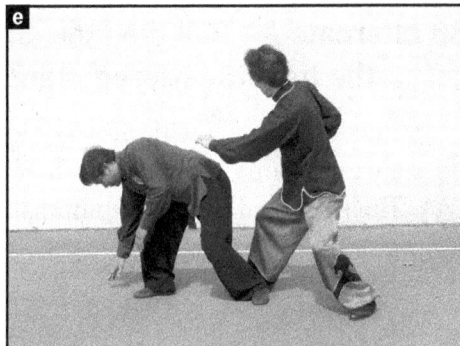

38 alternate A - Pull the bow. Shoot the tiger. Scattered stance.

If he kicks at you with his right leg, sidestep and scoop up his kick with your right arm. Then punch downward to his southern region.

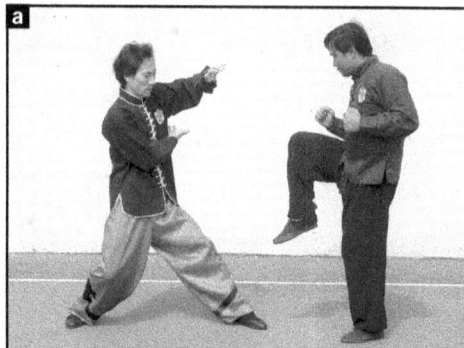

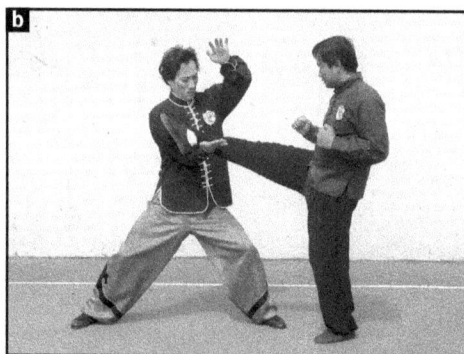

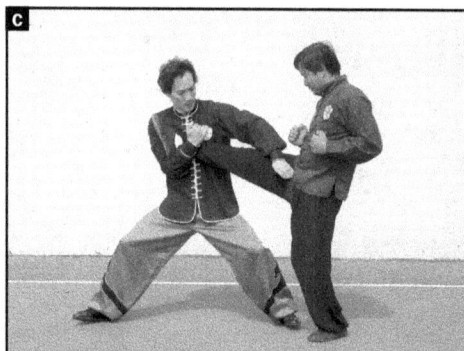

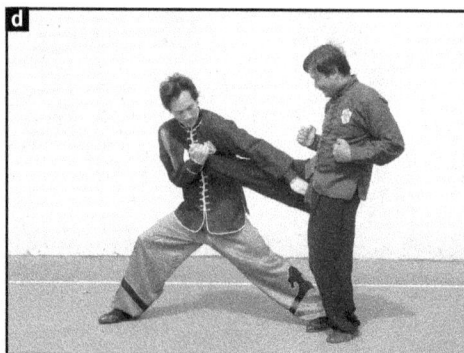

166

38 alternate B

Alternatively, after scooping up his
leg, you may strike him in his thigh.

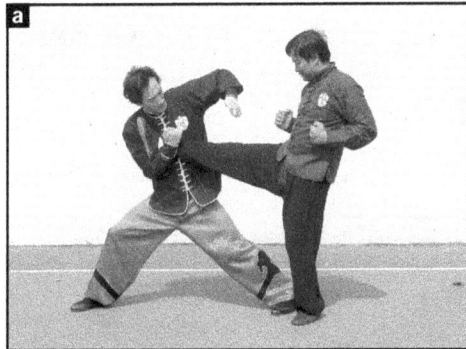

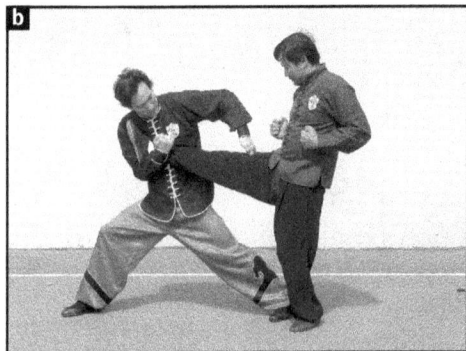

39 - Hero stands on one leg.
     Strike the tiger.

As he attempts to strike you with his right hand, parry downward with your left hand, and raise your left knee to strike him in the midsection.

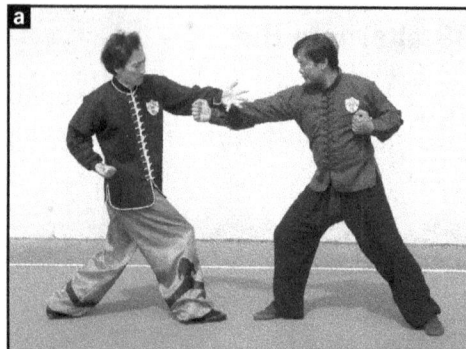

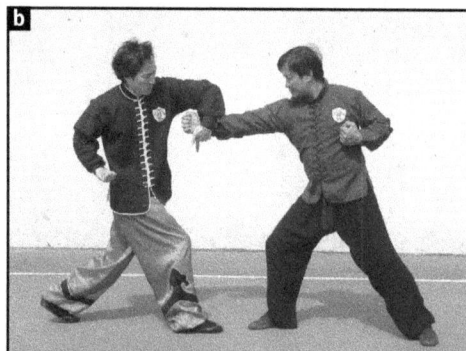

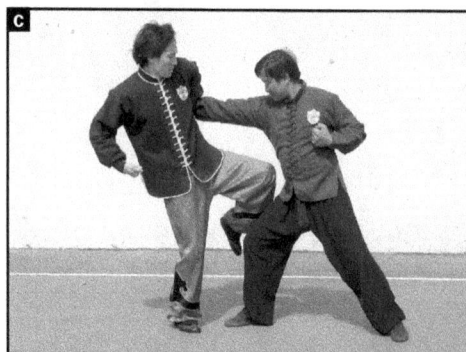

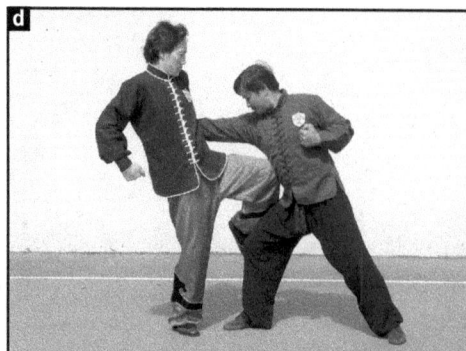

39 continued

Follow this with a right knuckle strike to his head.

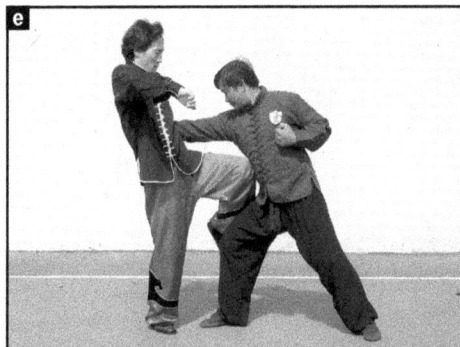

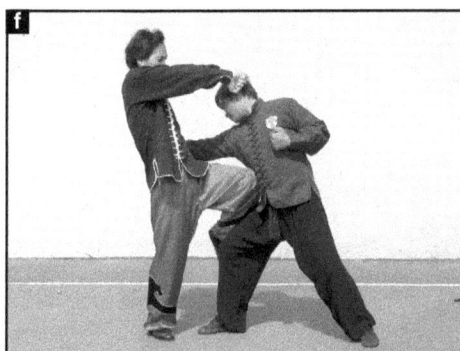

40A - Step back. Thrust palm.

For posture #40, some will say that the palm thrust has an application as a strike to the throut, while others will see all of #40A and #40B as simply a closing bow.

Either way of thinking about this move is acceptable.

Names of Movements of Shaolin #8

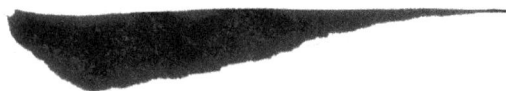

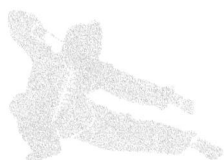

Names of Movements of Shaolin #8

1   Immortal shakes his clothes.
Step forward.
Double matching fists.

2   (Left) pulling hand.
Angled (side) step.
Advance with a (right) cutting palm in a right bow stance.

3

   3A)   Step back. (Right leg up, left palm.)
   3B)   "Uppercut to the groin" (right) palm strike.

4

   4A)   Step forward (Left cat stance).
            Lift hands. (Left palm strike).
   4B)   Sit in horse stance. Block and strike. (Right fist strike).

5

   5A)   (Raise the right leg.)
   5B)   Stamp the foot.
            Tangling hand.
            Step forward.
            Press and strike.

6   Wipe off the hand.
Strike with the palm.
Horse stance.

7   Back sweep.
Slap the ground.
Flying sand.

8

8A)   Double kick.

8B)   Stand up.

         Block and strike.

9   Turn around.

         The willow tree sways with the blowing wind.

         Go through the heart elbow. ("Protect the heart" elbow.)

10

10A) Strike with the fist. (Backfist strike).

10B) Kick with the (right) leg.

10C) Forward stance. Block and strike. (Right fist).

11   Step forward.

         Uppercut palm strike to the groin.

12   Stamp the ground. Strike with the fist.

13   Tornado kick.

14   Goddess sprinkles the flowers.

15

15A) Green dragon turns the body. (Right palm strike).

15B) Sit in a horse stance. Block and strike. (Left fist).

16   Tai Mountain collapses on the head. Right bow stance.

17

17A) Continuous flying kick.

17B) Fall down to the ground.

         Double pushing palms in a right bow stance.

18

18A) Back sweep.

18B) Hawk grabs the shoulder. (Right palm strike).

18C) Block and strike. (Left fist strike).

19   Left and right, flip the hands upward.
Crane stance. (Single leg).

20   Turn around.
Right leg flying lotus kick.

21   Come down to the ground.
Double wind strikes the ears. Right bow stance.

22   Twist stance.
Thrust to the groin with both fists.

23

    23A) Flipping hand (fist), left thrust kick.
    23B) Right toe kick.
    23C) Double pushing palm.

24   Back sweep.

25   Slap the ground.
Flying sand.

26   Double kick.

27   Come down to the ground.
Right bow stance.
Block and strike. (Left blocks and right fist strikes.)

28   Steal a step.
Wipe off the hand.
Block and strike.

29   Turn around.
Sit in a horse stance.
Block and strike.

30
    30A)   Raise the right leg.
    30B)   Stamp the foot.
             Tangling hand.
             Step forward.
             Press and strike (fist).

31
             Double hooking hands.
             Kick to the face.

32
    32A)   Double uplifting hands.
             Flying kick.
    32B)   Come down to the ground in a left bow stance.
             Double pushing palms.

33
             Turn around and slap the ground with the palms in a cross-legged stance.

34
             Turn around.
             Pulling hand. (Left)
             Straight punch. (Right)

35
             Right kick.

36
    36A)   Right straight punch. Right bow stance.
    36B)   Left straight punch. Right bow stance.

37
             Tornado kick.

38
             Pull the bow.
             Shoot the tiger.
             Scattered stance.

39
             Hero stands on one leg.
             Strike the tiger.

40

40A) Step back. Thrust palm.
40B) Finishing posture.

Notes on the Names of the Movements in Shaolin #8

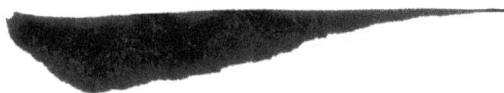

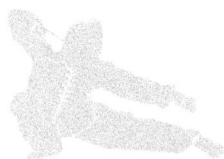

Notes on the Names of the Movements in Shaolin #8

Movement #1

"Double matching fists" could also have been translated as "paired fists" or "matching fists."

Movement #2

Note that the original Chinese does not say with which hand you are to pull with. I might add in left or right for clarity, and, in this case, you are to pull with the left hand and strike with the right palm.

Movement #3

Notice that the words in the original Chinese simply say "step back" and the hand motion is not described. When stepping out and striking with the edge of the right hand, the name would indicate that perhaps long ago, a practitioner would drop his right hand down and flick the hand up so as to attack the groin of the opponent.

Movement #4

For clarity I have added left and right because the original Chinese might be vague for someone unfamiliar with the form. It might also be a bit vague for someone even well-acquainted with the form.

Movement #5

For clarity in the photographs and for making the sequence of the form easier to follow, I added the name, ""Raise the right leg." I also did this for movement #30.

"Stamp the foot" could also have been translated as "stomp the foot." "Tangling" hand could have been translated as "trapping" or "controlling" hand. Notice that in the original Chinese, it only says "press and strike," and does not say to strike with the right palm.

Movement #9

The name "Willow tree sways with the blowing wind" is to indicate that you are to be soft and pliable as you do this movement. This is similar to the concept of "shao-lin" which means "young forest."

Movement #10

Notice again that the original Chinese writing does not say which arm or leg you are to strike with. It only describes the motion.

Movement #14

"Goddess sprinkles the flowers" could also have been translated as "Goddess spreads the flowers."

Movement #15

This could also have been translated as "Green dragon turns around."

Movement #16

The name of this movement indicates the force with which you are to strike with the right backfist.

Movement #17

Notice that the way the movements were grouped by number seems to be rather arbitrary. It would seem that sometimes, a double kick might have its own number, and the next movement will have its own number. Here, the double kick and the next move were grouped together.

Movement #18

Here, many movements seem to be grouped together under a single number. Sometimes, even an experienced Northern Shaolin practitioner will have difficulty in explaining why the names were grouped as such.

Movement #19

Although for these photos, I hold my left fist by my left side, some practitioners will hold their left hand in the crane's beak position and pull the left arm back and upward. Either method is acceptable.

Movement #20

The original Chinese only says "right lotus kick" and does not indicate that this is a jumping kick.

Movement #23

Notice that someone else might have used separate numbers for these movements. I have separated certain movements by using hyphenated numbers, although the original Chinese writings group them together. This is a convention I adopted to make the form more clear, but at the same time, I tried to remain true to the old Chinese numbering method. (Note: This may change in the future, i.e. our other works may not follow this convention.)

Movements #24 and #25

Similarly, these movements were earlier grouped together. Why they were separated here is not clear to me. But the photos and the showing of the sequence of the form will still be clear to the reader.

Movement #30

Notice that movement #30 has the same words as movement #5. Although the words are the same, movement #5 ends with a right palm strike and movement #30 ends with a right fist strike.

Movement #35

This could have been called "Ten" character kick or "Cross" kick, since this movement is a right leg heel kick and a left fist strike.

Movement #36

As usual, the original Chinese will say "Left, right straight punch" but I changed it to "Right and left straight punch" since that is the order in which it is done in the form. Typically, the Chinese writing will usually say "left, right" no matter what the order of the movements are, because (as I've been told) it sounds better in Chinese to say "left and right" instead of "right and left." This is similar to English speaking people using the words "up and down" instead of "down and up," no matter which way the movement actually occurred.

Movement #38

"Scattered" stance could have been translated as "collapsed" stance.

Movement #39

The "Hero stands on one leg" name corresponds to the stamping of the right foot as it sets on the ground, followed by the lifting of the left leg. The "Strike the tiger" name refers to the striking motion of the hands.

Names of Movements in Chinese Calligraphy

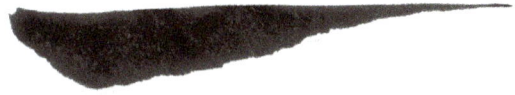

第 八 路

拔 步

少 林 拳

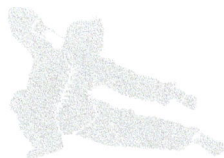

一、仙人彈衣上步對拳

二、摟手斜步右切掌

三、撤步撩陰掌

四、撩手上步坐馬架打式

五、震足纏手上步壓打

六、脫手撐掌坐馬式

七、後掃堂拍地飛沙

八、二起腿直立架打式

九、回身迎風擺柳窩心肘

十、扎拳踢腳弓步架打式

十一、上步撩陰掌

十二、恨地栽錘

十三、旋風腿

十四、偷步仙女散花

十五、青龍轉身坐馬架打式

188

十六、泰山壓頂右弓式

十七、連環飛踢落地雙推拳

十八、後掃堂鷹子抓肩架打式

十九、左右撩手獨立勢

二十、轉身右擺蓮腿

二一、落地雙風貫耳拳

二二、拗步分插錘

二三、挑手左蹬右踢雙推掌

二四、後掃堂腿

二五、拍地飛沙

二六、二起腿

二七、落地弓步架打式

二八、偷步脫手架打式

二九、轉身坐馬架打式

三十、震足纏手上步壓打

Acknowledgements

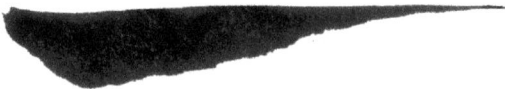

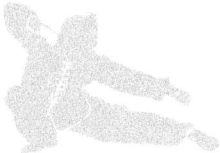

Acknowledgements

Let us again acknowledge the usual suspects.

Albert Koo helped with the preliminary translation, which was then fine-tuned by Master Paul Eng. Master Paul Eng, as usual, has graced the cover of the book with his fine calligraphy.

He then passed the ball to Mrs. Hsiu Fong Hao, wife of Mr. Tien Shou Hao, who showed her patience and skill by doing the calligraphy in the final section of the book. Any questions about the calligraphy should be referred to them, as there were a few characters which I was unsure of, like... all of them.

I must also mention our usual team of Mr. Remus Barraca, who helped in the applications section and Phillip Wong, who took all the photos again, and again, and again. The work was edited by Brennan Pelosi. Lastly, for the team, Robert Tichacek kicked it off, and Mr. Bruce Hopkins, the digital artist, brought it home.